Assessing Health Care Reform

Committee on Assessing
Health Care Reform Proposals

Marilyn J. Field, Kathleen N. Lohr,
and Karl D. Yordy, Editors

Division of Health Care Services

INSTITUTE OF MEDICINE

NATIONAL ACADEMY PRESS
Washington, D.C. 1993

NATIONAL ACADEMY PRESS • 2101 Constitution Avenue, N.W. • Washington, D.C. 20418

This study was supported by the W. K. Kellogg Foundation endowment fund.

Library of Congress Catalog Card No. 93-84089
International Standard Book Number 0-309-04926-1

Additional copies of this report are available from:

National Academy Press
2101 Constitution Avenue, NW
Washington, DC 20418

B150

Printed in the United States of America
First Printing, April 1993
Second Printing, October 1993
Third Printing, March 1994

The serpent has been a symbol of long life, healing, and knowledge among almost all cultures and religions since the beginning of recorded history. The image adopted as a logotype by the Institute of Medicine is based on a relief carving from ancient Greece, now held by the Staatlichemuseen in Berlin.

COMMITTEE ON ASSESSING
HEALTH CARE REFORM PROPOSALS

WALTER J. McNERNEY (*Chair*),* Professor of Health Policy and Consultant, J. L. Kellogg Graduate School of Management, Northwestern University, Chicago

LONNIE R. BRISTOW,* Private practice of internal medicine, San Pablo, California

DON E. DETMER,* Professor of Surgery and Vice President for Health Sciences, University of Virginia, Charlottesville

CLAIRE M. FAGIN,* Professor, School of Nursing, University of Pennsylvania, Philadelphia

JEROME H. GROSSMAN,* Chairman and Chief Executive Officer, The New England Medical Center, Boston

MARGARET C. HEAGARTY,* Director of Pediatrics, Harlem Hospital Center, and Professor of Pediatrics, College of Physicians & Surgeons, Columbia University, New York, New York

JOSEPH P. NEWHOUSE,* John D. MacArthur Professor of Health Policy and Management, Division of Health Policy Research and Education, Harvard University, Boston

EDWARD B. PERRIN,* Professor and Chairman, Department of Health Services, University of Washington, School of Public Health and Community Medicine, Seattle

GARY TISCHLER, Professor and Chairman, Department of Psychiatry and Biobehavioral Sciences, University of California at Los Angeles, School of Medicine

REED V. TUCKSON, President, Charles R. Drew University of Medicine and Science, Los Angeles

---

*Member, Institute of Medicine

STUDY STAFF

Marilyn J. Field, Principal Staff Officer
Kathleen N. Lohr, Deputy Director, Division of Health Care Services
Karl D. Yordy, Director, Division of Health Care Services
Holly Dawkins, Research Assistant, Division of Health Care Services
Don Tiller, Administrative Assistant, Division of Health Care Services

Contents

Assessing
Health Care
Reform

Preamble

The United States appears to be on the verge of instituting significant reform of the financing and organization of personal health care services. President Clinton is committed to submitting a proposal for reform in the near future, and many alternative proposals have already been put forward. These proposals vary widely in philosophy and mechanics, even as they seek the common objectives of universal access to affordable care and better control of escalating costs.

Although many Institute members are—as individuals—closely associated with various of the current reform proposals, the Institute of Medicine (IOM) has not developed its own comprehensive plan for reform. The judgments needed to formulate such a comprehensive plan involve specific trade-offs among social and economic values that are more appropriately addressed by the political process. We believe, however, that the IOM can make a different kind of contribution to the debate by helping to establish a framework for assessing reform proposals *and* their implementation. This framework should clarify objectives, identify issues that proposals should address, distinguish between what should be expected and achieved in the short versus the long term, and direct attention to important but sometimes neglected questions about the organization and provision of health services.

To this end, the IOM appointed a subcommittee of its Board on Health Care Services to develop a brief report that would be useful to all who are developing or assessing options for reform and that would apply to most of the likely reform scenarios. In developing this report, the committee has drawn where possible on the prior work of the IOM,

1

whose independent committees of experts have addressed many relevant topics in previous reports. Although these earlier studies do not provide a "grand plan" for reform, they do yield a body of considered analyses and recommendations that can help shape particular elements of such a plan. The committee has, in addition, gone beyond existing IOM reports to provide its own judgments and recommendations on some issues that it considers essential to achieving the goals outlined below.

In very broad terms, the committee identified fundamental goals for health care reform as a starting point for its report. These goals are to:

- **maintain and improve health and well-being;**
- **make basic health coverage universal; and**
- **encourage the efficient use of limited resources.**

Furthermore, reforms should honor, whenever possible, the American preference for diversity and personal choice in arrangements for health services. Reform proposals should also acknowledge and emphasize the responsibility and accountability of individuals, health professionals, and society as a whole for improving health and well-being.

Health and well-being depend on many factors in addition to health care coverage and services. Because environmental, educational, and other activities also enable people to lead healthier lives, society increasingly has come to understand that reforms should seek to improve what the health care system achieves while minimizing the diversion of resources from these other beneficial activities.

Although there will be pressure on policymakers to look for quick results, significant progress on the goals identified above will require patience and commitment over many years. It is critical that reforms be structured and implemented in ways that make possible systematic learning and program revisions based on experience. The arrangements for health care are so complex and the implications of major reform so profound that it is unrealistic to act as if we will know all of the answers when implementation of a plan is begun. Many aspects of reform will evolve over a period of years. This evolution will, in fact, place a premium, first, on having good information on which to base an evaluation of results and, second, on the flexibility to respond to the evaluation and modify programs—thus our emphasis in this report on the importance of good data about health and health care. In addition to building on strong clinical and health systems information, successful reform will also require sensitivity to the individual and social values that underlie our approaches to health and health care.

In developing a framework for assessing health care reform, the committee has focused on five topics:

- extending access to health care;
- containing costs and improving value;
- assuring the quality of care;
- financing reform; and
- improving the infrastructure for effective change.

The first three topics relate closely to the fundamental goals for health care reform that the committee identified above. The last two topics address essential means for achieving those goals. The committee believes that any plan or proposal intended to bring about significant movement toward the goals should address each area, although the mix of responses and the trade-offs among objectives will vary according to the values of the decisionmakers.

The infrastructure component of this framework is, in the committee's view, particularly important. Many key decisionmakers will not be health care experts and may not fully appreciate why reform proposals should recognize the crucial links between policies to expand access, control costs, and assure quality, and policies to improve system governance and administration, knowledge development and its application, human and physical capital, and community-focused public health programs. These infrastructure improvements are essential to reform over the long term and can proceed in parallel with other aspects of reform; the committee would not want infrastructure needs to be used as an excuse to delay health care reform.

The committee has not addressed the complicated issues of long-term institutional or home care, not because these issues are unimportant but because they cannot be treated adequately in this short report. The financing and provision of long-term care deals, in particular, with assistance in the activities of daily living, and therefore requires attention to related issues of housing, social services, and transportation, as well as income support policies, estate preservation, and encouragement of continued voluntary efforts by spouses, other relatives, and friends. The burgeoning costs of the Medicaid program are heavily affected by long-term care expenses. The committee hopes that policymakers will also be able to focus on these concerns while health care reform for acute care services is being debated and implemented.

Finally, in this short document, the committee has focused on the kinds of issues that will particularly engage central policymakers in a direction-setting role. It has tried, nonetheless, to reflect the reality that health care is provided in thousands of local communities by tens of thousands of practitioners, administrators, and others working with real patients, families, and problems. The committee urges those developing reform proposals and making policy decisions to vigorously and continuously seek the experience and insights of those who work daily to maintain health, manage illness, and sustain dignity under circumstances that range from commonplace to desperate.

PREAMBLE

Key Statements

The fundamental goals for health care reform are to:

- maintain and improve health and well-being;
- make basic health coverage universal; and
- encourage the efficient use of limited resources.

Extending Access to Health Care

For many policymakers and citizens, the defining objective of health care reform is to create more uniform, secure, and effective access to health care and health insurance for the people of the United States. This focus is understandable. Millions of Americans are uninsured or otherwise lack reasonable access to health care. Millions more fear that an illness, an employer's decision to cut health benefits, or some other event beyond their control could deprive them of coverage. Even voluntary actions, for example, a job change, are increasingly constrained by concerns about continued health coverage. What was once perceived as largely a problem for low-income people is now a growing concern for middle-income people as well.

Just as the cost of medical care is a major problem for many Americans, high and increasing health care costs are a major obstacle to health care reform. It has, for instance, been argued that health care costs must be contained *before* major steps to extend health coverage can be undertaken. The committee believes that such a two-step reform strategy underestimates the foreseeable costs of not extending access, in particular, the extent to which the lack of universal health coverage produces costly distortions in the way care is provided and financed and in the decisions made by employers, employees, and others. These distortions include patient delays in getting needed care, "job lock" (which occurs when a worker refuses an otherwise better job because it does not include any or acceptable health benefits), and to cost-shifting (when providers try to recover costs related to charity care and underpayments from public payers through higher prices to private payers).

The committee, nonetheless, expects that expanding health coverage will add to total health care spending—both public and private—in the near term. Although a phased-in strategy for broad reform—including a phased-in approach to improved access—is reasonable, such an approach should include early steps to achieve broader and more predictable health coverage. Expanded access should not become a second-stage contingency.

The primary barriers to access stressed in most reform proposals are financial—in particular, absent, inadequate, or unreliable health insurance. Proposals should also be grounded in a realistic understanding that access to effective health services is more than a matter of money. Other barriers to access also require attention.

BARRIERS TO ACCESS

Many obstacles can stand in the way of the timely use of effective health services. These obstacles include

- financial barriers, as noted above;
- distance from primary, secondary, and tertiary medical services, a problem exacerbated by transportation limitations;
- lack of education, language barriers, unsafe neighborhoods, and other nonmedical problems;
- deficiencies in the structure and functioning of the health care system, including the general lack of coordinated approaches to service delivery and provider payment levels that in some programs (notably Medicaid) may be too low to secure adequate access to care for beneficiaries; and
- shortfalls in our knowledge of how clinical care, the community and workplace environments, and individual social, cultural, and biological characteristics interact to affect health status and the use of health services.

To the extent that health care reform helps to reduce these barriers, it can allow more people to improve their health and well-being by using the right medical services at the right time. No one, however, should expect such reform either to solve all health-related problems or to address the sources of these problems equally. For some problems, such as cocaine addiction in pregnant women, no effective medical therapies exist. For other problems, such as injuries and deaths due to domestic and neighborhood violence, nonmedical policies and programs that focus on issues such as job creation, education, and crime control may do more than medical programs to improve health and well-being. One reason for bringing the growth in health care spending more in line—even if only marginally—with growth in the rest of the economy is to free resources for these kinds of programs. In general, a long-term commitment to the objectives of health care reform requires a prudent appreciation of both the promise and limits of health care reform for achieving better health outcomes.

FINANCIAL ACCESS

Principles

On both philosophical and practical grounds, **the committee believes that an attack on financial barriers to health care should work from the basic, interrelated principles outlined below** (IOM 1991f, 1993a,b; NRC/IOM, 1992). Transforming these principles into legislation—and translating legislation into improved access to effective health services—will be exceedingly difficult for both political and technical reasons. Current opinion polls and hard experience point to a gap between the generous values that this nation broadly espouses and the narrower interests that we actively protect. These realities notwithstanding, the following principles are, in the committee's view, an appropriate foundation for health care reform. Some important practical implications and difficulties raised by these principles are discussed in the next section.

• **All or virtually all persons—whether employed or not, whether ill or well, whether old or young—must participate in a health benefits plan.** The plan may be a single nationwide program or one of several alternative public or private plans, but no one should need to depend on charity care or be allowed to stay uninsured while they are healthy.

   · Whether a single health plan or multiple plans are envisioned, **a uniform package of core or basic health benefits must be defined and periodically updated.** The package should include an array of services that are thought to be valuable in improving health and well-being. The committee also believes that individuals should be able—consistent with equity and other policy objectives—to purchase coverage to supplement the core package on a non-tax-favored basis.

   · If multiple health benefit plans are permitted, **policies should minimize barriers to initial and continued health coverage (e.g., waiting periods and restrictions on coverage for preexisting health problems) for those who move, change jobs, become ill, start or stop receiving public assistance, or face similar changed circumstances.** Otherwise, such barriers will undermine both access to appropriate health care and labor market mobility.

   · **Requirements that individuals share in the cost of health coverage and health services should not create barriers to needed care for low income individuals,** although administrative practicality will limit the degree to which deductibles, copayments, and similar cost-sharing mechanisms can vary by income. Certain services, such as selected preventive services, might be exempted altogether from cost-sharing provisions.

   · To reduce incentives for health benefit plans to compete for healthy individuals and avoid the ill, **the payments received by health plans (from governments, employers, or other sources) should be adjusted to reflect important differences in the distribution of low-risk and high-risk individuals across health plans.** Some plans may also receive additional support for intensive outreach programs for special populations such as low-income mothers and children.

   · **Correspondingly, what individuals pay for health coverage should not be linked to their health status (past or anticipated), age, gender, occupation, or similar factors.** Thus, what an individual pays into the system for health coverage may differ from what is paid out to a health plan for enrolling that individual. Some argue that it is fairer and more efficient to link individuals' payments for coverage to their risk of incurring expenses, but, on balance, the committee believes that such discrimination in the cost of coverage is a divisive and highly imperfect way of achieving greater efficiency in the financing, use, or provision of health services.

Practical Implications

This discussion highlights only a few of the more prominent implications of the above principles. **First,** if coverage is to be universal, the healthy and the well off must share the cost of covering the ill and the poor. This is not simply a matter of philanthropy but a reflection of our common and lifelong vulnerability to illness and disability—to moving from the category of well to ill. However, to the extent that people are divided into multiple, separate financing arrangements (or risk pools) such as employee groups, a broad sharing of the costs of protection against medical expenses becomes more administratively and politically complex. As recommended earlier, requirements that individuals share in the cost of health coverage and health services should provide for some adjustment by income, within the bounds of administrative feasibility. Again, the details of a benefit package may be left to administrative agencies or perhaps a special commission, but a reform proposal must set forth basic criteria and procedures to be followed.

Second, any proposal that involves multiple health benefit plans requires methods and mechanisms for (1) distributing payments to health plans and (2) augmenting any individual payments for coverage with contributions from employers, governments, or others that are adequate to cover appropriate, efficient care to the specific mix of more and less healthy individuals who select any particular plan. Without such adjustments, which may involve government, employers, or specially created organizations such as purchasing cooperatives, health plans will face strong incentives to market only to the well and to discourage enrollment by the less healthy. Unfortunately, strategies to adjust payments to reflect risk selection are not yet technically or practically adequate, although progress is being made. The more a reform proposal includes other means to manage or compensate for risk selection, however, the lighter the burden will be on techniques for adjusting health plan payments.   Standardized benefit packages, some reinsurance provisions, and monitoring for abusive health plan marketing and management practices are examples of such means (IOM, 1993b).

Third, a provision for core or standardized benefits based on effectiveness implies the need for explicit processes and criteria for defining and updating such benefits that build on the best scientific evidence and professional judgment available.   Some of the most politically sensitive questions any reform proposal must answer are: who will define and update the basic package and determine any restrictions on supplemental coverage, what measures of effectiveness will be employed to include, exclude, or discontinue coverage for specific services, and what other criteria for inclusion will be employed?   The stakes involved in benefit design are very high for specific categories of health care providers and patients. Formidable difficulties face any effort to establish a structure that is reasonably accountable to the public, reasonably insulated against pressures from narrow interest groups to expand excessively the core package of benefits, and reasonably feasible to initiate and sustain over time.   Points four through seven below and the discussion of core and supplemental benefits in the cost containment section of this report all underscore this point.   Again, defining basic benefits will present policymakers with many difficult problems.

Fourth, at this stage, evidence for the effectiveness of a great many services—including many that are widely believed to be effective and that are generally covered by public and private health plans—simply does not exist (IOM, 1992b). Many (perhaps most) judgments about what services are appropriate or—more stringently—essential will have a considerable subjective component that should be acknowledged. One element of subjectivity relates to expert judgment in the absence of evidence; another involves differences between experts and patients (or among patients) in judgments about what outcomes are important. It will be expensive and time-consuming to increase our base of scientific knowledge and bring professional judgment systematically to bear on the question of what care is effective for the great range of individual health problems. Thus, linking a core benefit package to services of demonstrated effectiveness and value to patients will be an incremental process.[1] Initially, many services of undocumented effectiveness would need to be covered to reflect patient, practitioner, and community perceptions of what care is appropriate. As our knowledge base expands (as discussed in the section on infrastructure), that should change.

Fifth, whether the package of core benefits should be relatively narrow or broad will be a major point of contention as the objective of expanding access competes with policymakers' efforts to limit the cost of making the basic package available to those now uninsured. **To limit inequities in access, the committee believes that the core package or standard plan needs to be reasonably comprehensive.**

Sixth, if the core package is defined narrowly (e.g., it omits coverage for outpatient prescription drugs and mental health services) to reduce the cost to government and employers of subsidizing it, then supplemental benefits will become more important to many individuals. Purchase of such benefits, however, will be difficult for lower income individuals, and even employer-paid supplemental coverage may be a limited blessing if it increases individual tax liability. If the core package of benefits is a "bare bones" one, then the committee

---

[1]The difference between a benefit package as traditionally understood by insurers and a benefit package as understood by those proposing effectiveness-based coverage needs further examination. Given the difficulty consumers now have in understanding health insurance contract language, it is hard to imagine they would understand a health insurance contract or contract addendum with hundreds of pages of fine print spelling out such things as whether a coronary artery bypass graft would be covered for an individual with mild chronic stable angina who has single-vessel disease and a negative exercise electrocardiogram and who is not a candidate for percutaneous transluminal cutaneous angioplasty. It is even harder to imagine such contracts in the context of health plans that would compete (and be evaluated by consumers) on the basis of nonuniform benefit packages that differed at this level of detail. It may be more useful conceptually to treat most condition-specific coverage limitations not as part of the benefits package itself but rather as essential elements in interpreting and applying coverage. The specifics of such coverage limits should be made public—unlike the criteria now used by many health plans for utilization management. Whether these criteria are part of the benefits contract, an addendum, or a coverage administration manual, an average citizen may be dazed by the detailed specifications of what care will and will not be covered.

recommends that supplemental benefits for selected services be tax-favored.

Seventh, reforms that provide for basic and supplemental benefits imply additional procedures and methods for relating the two kinds of benefits and monitoring both. The aim is to ensure that the availability and marketing of the supplemental benefits do not seriously subvert the equity and effectiveness objectives sought through the definition of a basic benefit package and do not unduly complicate the evaluation of competitive health plans with different supplemental coverage. This may require that supplemental benefits be priced separately and purchasable either from the plan providing the basic benefit package or separately. Depending on the way core and supplemental benefits are structured in the context of a comprehensive plan for health care reform, adverse selection might make supplemental benefits unworkable except perhaps for those provided across-the-board by employers to all their employees.

Eighth, a provision for standardized benefits implies a process for defining benefits that applies to health maintenance organizations and other network health plans as well as fee-for-service settings, assuming that a reform proposal accommodates both. A related issue is how patients should be informed about health plan policies that constrain access to certain generally covered services, for example, formularies that limit access to many drugs or staffing criteria that restrict the numbers and kinds of practitioners available to provide mental health services. The varied opportunities for health plans to restrict access may, in turn, imply the need for some system to monitor that covered services are reasonably available from health plans and not just pro forma promises in health plan brochures. For example, if patients face long delays in getting a particular service in the basic benefit package because their network health plan has deliberately hired or contracted with too few providers of that service, does the plan at some point fall out of compliance with basic benefit requirements? The design of a reform proposal should include some guidance on such questions, even if most details are left to implementers.

Ninth, because reforms, once adopted, cannot just be assumed to be successful in meeting their objectives, policymakers need to monitor changes in access over time. A recent IOM report (IOM, 1993a) contains specific recommendations on this point, and the discussion of information and research issues in this report is also relevant.

Tenth, if a reform proposal would continue employment-based health benefits, the committee believes that **the Employee Retirement Income Security Act must be significantly amended and strengthened.** The discretion now accorded self-insured health plans, on the one hand, and state insurance regulators, on the other, should be rationalized and, in a number of areas, circumscribed. Critical coverage, funding, and other health plan features should be made more consistent across health plans, more reliable and predictable over time, and less of a barrier to the continuity of health care and job mobility.

More generally, the current relationships between public and private programs and state and federal policy with respect to health benefits will require considerable rethinking and realignment. **Health care reform proposals that aim to provide universal coverage and control costs should define the role of existing public sector health care coverage or service programs such as Medicare, Medicaid, the Department of Veterans Affairs health system, public health services, and various federal block grants to states and communities.** Even if reform proposals do not directly encompass the beneficiaries of such programs, they should be clear about how those massive public programs ought to tackle their own serious access and expenditures issues. Moreover, those parts of any reform effort intended to extend insurance coverage to the uninsured must also address the problems of the poor and medically needy who may (or may not), on any given day, be eligible for or enrolled in Medicaid.

The current structure of the federal–state Medicaid program is already the subject of much dissatisfaction independent of the agitation for health care reform. Several options exist for Medicaid. They include retaining Medicaid's focus on the medically indigent but improving program policymaking and operations; expanding it to enroll individuals not covered by employment-based plans; modifying the program by moving the elderly long-term care portions to Medicare; limiting the program to long-term care; or abolishing it altogether and covering everyone not eligible for Medicare or employment-based coverage under a single health program. Neither this committee nor other IOM groups have systematically examined these approaches; thus, the committee takes no position on them. The committee emphasizes, however, the importance of thoroughly rethinking the program's role and structure.

Assessing Access Provisions of Reform Proposals

Whatever their specific philosophy and approach, **reform proposals should be sufficiently detailed that policymakers and others can understand and evaluate six key dimensions of the reform strategy.** These dimensions are:

• The processes and criteria that would be used to define the core benefit package, including how they would take into account health outcomes, financial constraints, community values, patient preferences, and scientific evidence; how the package would be revised to take changing technology or other factors into account; how the benefit package would relate to prepaid or capitated delivery systems; and what kind of role would be envisioned for coverage that individuals or their employers could purchase to supplement the core benefits.
• The processes and policies that would be adopted to discourage or overcome biased risk selection and discrimination against higher-risk and higher-cost individuals.
• The restrictions, if any, that would be placed on the free choice by individuals of health practitioners and providers.
• The provisions that would be needed to minimize disruptions in continuity of care that could arise from employers, governments, or other purchasers changing the health plans they sponsor, from individuals changing jobs, or from turnover in the practitioners associated with particular health plans.
• The degree to which geographical or employer-based variations in the cost of coverage would be allowed or limited.
• The ways special categories of individuals such as foreign tourists and undocumented foreign workers would be treated.

MORE THAN FINANCIAL ACCESS

Because improved access and health status are key goals of health care reform, and because impediments to the achievement of these goals are not just financial, proposals to extend health insurance coverage should define where coordination is needed with other public and private programs that target these nonfinancial barriers. Such programs will include:

• broad **public health and health education initiatives** that help people understand how to take care of their health, use health care services appropriately, and seek healthful environments in the home, the workplace, and the community;
• efforts to structure health care services, systems, and financing to more effectively reach **special populations** such as residents of inner city and rural areas, high-risk mothers and children, frail elderly persons, homeless and migrant groups, and those with certain health problems such as AIDS, substance abuse, and severe mental illness;
• programs to recruit and train (or retrain) health care practitioners to support **expanded access to primary and preventive services**, especially in areas where such services are already in short supply;
• **clinical and health services research** that provides a better knowledge base on which to construct education, health promotion, and special outreach activities; and
• vigorous, well-financed programs of **quality assurance and health services research** to help protect against potential unwanted side effects of health system bureaucracies (both public and private) and cost containment efforts.

These programs, in turn, will require bridges to nonmedical programs and policies that focus directly on the many social and other problems that particularly burden some populations. Although health programs are not the main avenue for tackling such issues, health workers may involve themselves with problems as diverse as homelessness, inner city and rural transportation deficits, and domestic violence.

For no special population is concern more acute than for children and pregnant women, especially those who are at high risk either medically or socioeconomically. **Reform proposals should include specific provisions for these groups; that is, they should cover all or virtually all the cost of services that are critical to the health and well-being of these groups.** For children, these services include routine immunizations, well-child care, and routine dental care. For pregnant women and women of childbearing age, benefits should include prenatal diagnosis and care and family planning services. For those at highest risk, provision for nutritional support and maternity outreach will be necessary (IOM, 1985, 1992d,e), in addition to services covered under the basic benefit package.

Public sector health and social networks for disadvantaged children and high-risk pregnant women are, for the foreseeable future, essential to ensure their access to these kinds of services. Under some circumstances, comprehensive, multidisciplinary, community-based centers can be more effective in serving these populations than free-standing private practices, because the sociomedical problems of these individuals are often greater than a single office-based practice can accommodate (IOM 1992d,e). The special resource needs of such comprehensive centers for disadvantaged children and pregnant women should be recognized if they are to offer effective services.

Also, health plan features designed with the middle class in mind may prove to be significant obstacles to obtaining appropriate, effective, and timely care for those with low levels of income and education. For example, some managed care plans now decline to pay for more than 24 hours of hospital care following normal childbirth, thus reducing the opportunity to monitor newborns in the critical first one or two days after birth and to teach new mothers how to care for their babies.

Such policies, as well as requirements for advance approval of hospitalization and similar cost containment policies in private and public health plans, should be studied to determine whether they impede the use of appropriate or effective health services, particularly by special populations. The same call for research also applies to the complicated administrative structures that cut across or link coverage under public and private programs for the elderly, the poor, and other groups. Even for the college educated, health plan rules and procedures can be confusing and discouraging, and they also demoralize health care practitioners.

A challenge for health care reform is to minimize bureaucratic complexity and to assist people in negotiating the structural and procedural complexity that remains. Such efforts will supplement quality assurance and research programs and help to identify and remedy both financial and nonfinancial barriers to appropriate care.

EXTENDING ACCESS TO HEALTH CARE

Key Statements

All or virtually all persons—whether employed or not, whether ill or well, whether old or young—must participate in a health benefits plan.

Whether a single plan or multiple plans are envisioned, a uniform package of core or basic health benefits must be defined and periodically updated. The package should include an array of services that are thought to be valuable in improving health and well-being. To limit inequities in access, the core package or standard plan needs to be reasonably comprehensive.

If multiple health benefit plans are permitted, policies should minimize barriers to initial and continued health coverage (such as waiting periods and restrictions on coverage for preexisting health problems) for those who move, change jobs, become ill, start or stop receiving public assistance, or face similar changed circumstances.

Requirements that individuals share in the cost of health coverage and health services should not create barriers to needed care for low income individuals.

To reduce incentives for health plans to compete for healthy individuals and avoid the ill, the payments received by health plans (from governments, employers, or other sources) should be adjusted to reflect important differences in the distribution of low-risk and high-risk individuals across health plans.

Correspondingly, what individuals pay for health coverage should not be linked to their health status (past or anticipated), age, gender, occupation, or similar factors. Thus, what an individual pays into the system for health coverage may differ from what is paid out to a health plan for enrolling that individual.

The Employee Retirement Income Security Act must be significantly amended and strengthened to rationalize and circumscribe the discretion now accorded self-insured health plans, on the one hand, and state insurance regulators, on the other. Critical coverage, funding, and other health plan features should be made more consistent across health plans, more reliable and predictable over time, and less of a barrier to continuity of health care and job mobility.

Health care reform proposals should define the role of existing public sector health care coverage or service programs such as Medicare, Medicaid, the Department of Veterans Affairs health system, public health services, and various federal block grants to states and communities.

Reform proposals should include specific provisions for benefits that cover all or virtually all the cost of services that are critical to the health and well-being of children and mothers, especially those at high risk.

Proposals to extend health insurance should define where coordination is needed with other public and private programs that target nonfinancial barriers to improved access and health status.

Because reforms, once adopted, cannot just be assumed to be successful in meeting their objectives, policymakers need to monitor changes in access over time.

Containing Health Care Costs

Given the many pressing demands on finite national resources and the rapid increase in the share of those resources devoted to health care, policymakers, business leaders, and ordinary citizens must be concerned with both the country's high absolute level of health care spending and its rapid rate of growth relative to the overall economy. As noted in the preceding section, cost concerns have been a major obstacle to efforts to expand access to health care for those who are now uninsured or underinsured. High health care costs are also a major contributor to growing anxiety among the middle class about the adequacy and continued availability of their health coverage.

COSTS IN CONTEXT

To serve health and access as well as cost containment objectives, **policies to limit the rate of cost escalation need to be grounded in the concepts of**:

- **value—how health care spending relates to the achievement of desired outcomes;**
- **affordability—how health care spending relates to individual and societal resources; and**
- **equity—how the financing and distribution of health services affects different groups.**

21

Further, to be sustainable, cost management tools and monitoring structures should encourage and emphasize individual, professional, and organizational accountability.   Detailed efforts to regulate prices, services, and other aspects of day-to-day health care delivery run two major risks. First, some health care practitioners and providers, health plans, and consumers may be preoccupied with manipulating the system rather than achieving more efficient and effective health services. Second, such manipulation may inspire ever more complex and voluminous rules that would ultimately defy sensible management or compliance by even the most well-intentioned participants. The current balance between delegation and regulation generates considerable tension and dissatisfaction, but some disagreement about the probable costs and benefits of any particular balance appears inevitable.

ELEMENTS OF A STRATEGY

As explained in the Preamble, the committee has not developed a comprehensive proposal for health care reform.   It also has not formulated a comprehensive cost containment strategy to reduce the rate of increases in health care costs. One reason is that evidence about the effectiveness of specific tools supports a rather cautious view about their prospects for significantly limiting the rate of increase in health care costs or even achieving some "once-and-for-all" savings. Reforms should not overlook opportunities for such savings (and the associated shift to a lower trajectory of cost escalation), but they should avoid overselling strategies of modest or unproved effectiveness. (For reviews of the literature on the impact of cost containment strategies, see CBO, 1992a, 1992b; EBRI, 1991; IOM, 1989b, 1993b; Jencks and Schieber, 1991; Newhouse, 1992; Thorpe, 1992.)

Moreover, although some individual committee members had strong philosophical views about managed competition and other relatively sweeping prescriptions for controlling health care costs, the committee did not reach consensus on such prescriptions as part of this particular effort. For policymakers and the public at large, however, the next few months will bring an intense effort to forge, from contending views, an effective consensus about short-term and long-term strategies to reduce the rate of increase in health care costs and help finance expanded access.

The remainder of this section briefly describes the elements of a cost containment strategy on which the committee focused and then discusses certain other options. The next section considers some of the questions that would need to be resolved in moving from general to specific policies.

Specific Elements

The committee agreed that several specific elements should have a role in a strategy for health care reform. These elements focus, for the most part, on the link between resource use and health outcomes, and they include:

• **Movement toward provider payment methods that encourage efficiency and economy in the provision of health services as well as quality of care and good outcomes.** Examples include payments partially based on an episode of illness (rather than individual services) and capitated payments to health plans (Newhouse, 1989), but the committee encourages experimentation (rather than commitment to a single approach). To avoid incentives for underservice to more seriously ill individuals, per case, capitated, and similar kinds of payments to providers or health plans should be adjusted to reflect the risk presented by a patient or health plan member. As noted earlier in this report, no fully satisfactory set of risk adjusters now exists.

• **Some cost-sharing by most patients** (e.g., deductibles, coinsurance, premiums). Patients should be motivated to weigh the costs of specific services and health plan options against their perceived benefits. Again, as noted previously, cost-sharing requirements for those with low incomes or high expenses should not constitute a barrier to needed care.

• **Better information on the price, quality, and expected outcomes of medical services** (see the section on infrastructure for further discussion). Such information should be presented in forms that are useful and timely (e.g., provided prior to decisions about care) for ordinary patients and consumers as well as for practitioners, managers, and policymakers. Strategies to increase consumer price sensitivity need to be balanced by actions to help people make informed decisions about complex issues even under often stressful circumstances (IOM, 1992b). To the extent, however, that better information leads sicker individuals to health plans or practitioners that can care more effectively for them, it will encourage adverse selection and put more pressure on the risk-adjusted payment approaches discussed elsewhere in this report.

• **Methods for quality and utilization review that help practitioners, patients, and others learn how actual care conforms to criteria for appropriate care and why care varies in effectiveness and efficiency.** These methods should be as unobtrusive as is feasible and consistent with the entire set of structures and incentives included in a reform proposal (IOM, 1989b, 1992b).

• **A tax cap that limits the amount of employer-paid health benefits excluded from individual taxable income.** The intent is to increase individual and employer sensitivity to the actual cost of different health plans, improve tax equity, and provide some revenues to help finance reforms (IOM, 1993b).

• **Further movement to standardize many administrative practices and eliminate many costs associated with the immense diversity of current billing, payment, audit, reporting, and other practices.**

Implementation of the above elements—particularly the first and second—should reduce some of the strain placed on the health care system by reducing the demand for care. It should simultaneously encourage informed evaluation of health care options so that reductions in demand are focused on care of marginal value. On balance, however, empirical evidence suggests that although the above strategies may produce some savings, they are not likely to be strong instruments for reducing the underlying rate of increase in health care costs (IOM, 1989b, 1993b).

Elements Not Mentioned

Some omissions from the above list of elements warrant comment. These omissions include managed competition, global budgets, health planning, and clinical practice guidelines.

The committee notes a strategy that is frequently promoted as a centerpiece of health care reform: "managed competition." Most versions of this strategy call for a regulated system of competition among health plans that limit coverage to care provided by restricted networks of practitioners and providers, for example, staff-model health maintenance organizations that rely on salaried physicians. Members of the committee disagree about whether a patient's choice of provider must be relinquished to contain costs, and they doubt that managed competition is feasible outside major metropolitan areas. Furthermore, empirical evidence about the cost containment effects of managed competition is essentially nonexistent because the full strategy has not been implemented. These reservations notwithstanding, the committee members agree that well-managed, "seamless" systems that integrate an array of medical services can improve the quality and efficiency of care.

The committee's list of cost containment measures also omits any reference to two other oft-mentioned strategies: a global limit or cap on health care spending and price and wage controls. The committee recognizes that budgets and caps may be essential or useful for some segments of the health care system, most obviously for government spending (including revenues lost through tax breaks for private spending). The committee, however, as a matter of philosophy, believes that individuals should be free to spend their after-tax dollars on health care or health insurance. Such freedom is inconsistent with a collectively determined and imposed limit on total spending. When, however, private choices affect the cost of the basic program, policymakers may consider limiting certain choices. An example would be discouraging the purchase of supplemental insurance designed to cover basic program deductibles and copayments; such coverage might erode the effectiveness of patient cost sharing as an incentive for lower health care utilization.

With respect to price and wage controls specifically, the committee recognizes the attraction of short-term price and wage controls (1) to achieve short-term savings that can be used to extend coverage to the uninsured, (2) to limit cost increases until longer term reforms begin to achieve results, or (3) to supplement long-term strategies, such as managed competition, that may not by themselves be sufficient to limit cost increases. Some committee members, however, doubt the practicality and desirability of even short-term price controls. They cite: the possibility that increased service volume will offset a freeze on unit prices; the complexity of determining what services, settings, and providers will be subject to the cap; the unfairness of subjecting, for example, janitors and food service workers in the health sector to wage controls when their peers in other sectors are unaffected; and the potential for black markets to arise for some services. Another worry is that short-term controls might undermine longer term reforms by discouraging organizational flexibility and innovation and failing to reward efficient practitioners and providers.

At a more specific level, the committee's list of elements of a cost containment strategy mentions neither health planning nor clinical practice guidelines. The former has risen and fallen in favor among policymakers (IOM, 1989b, 1993b) whereas the latter has only recently been promoted as a tool for cost containment. Health planning is cited in this report's discussion of infrastructure as one option for influencing the supply, distribution, and kinds of physical capital to meet a variety of policy objectives. A related discussion focuses on health workforce planning, in particular, the need to increase the proportion of primary care physicians who provide the preventive, primary care, and gatekeeping services that many reform proposals emphasize as means of increasing efficiency in health care delivery.

Clinical practice guidelines are also discussed later in this report as an element of strategies to improve quality of care. With respect to cost containment, policymakers should have reasonable expectations for practice guidelines (IOM, 1992b). Guidelines based on systematically evaluated scientific evidence and professional judgment currently apply to a relatively small proportion of all health services and specific patient problems, and such guidelines are expensive and time consuming to develop. Moreover, the net effect that guidelines may have on costs is hard to predict. Some guidelines, for example, those on proper management of pain, are likely to increase the use of some currently underused services; other guidelines are likely to discourage the use of currently overused services; in some cases, increased or decreased utilization will be offset by intended or unintended changes in care that has been or can be used in lieu of the target services; not uncommonly, guidelines are ignored.

MOVING FROM GENERAL TO SPECIFIC POLICIES

The design of specific policies to constrain costs and improve the value received for health care spending will require decisions about a large number of complex questions, many of which do not have obvious answers. Two particularly contentious questions involve the degree to which cost containment can work through market forces rather than regulation and the extent to which regional needs or wants can be accommodated. In general, the committee believes that reforms will require a **pragmatic mix of regulatory and market strategies and that some degree of local flexibility and discretion is desirable.** Further, a reform strategy oriented toward experimentation and learning in both the public and the private sectors holds more promise of long-term success than an approach that attempts to answer all key questions a priori. **Proposals should specify whether (and how) they would phase in certain components on a test-and-revise or compare-and-select basis.**

A few other prominent questions that proposals for health care reform should address are discussed below. The committee has a number of observations and a few specific recommendations regarding administrative costs, tax caps, cost sharing, benefit design, and biased risk selection.

Administrative Costs—and Benefits

Efforts to reduce administrative costs may, in some cases, conflict with efforts to collect more data for monitoring, educational, and other purposes. For example, as noted earlier, the committee believes that the continued growth of cost sharing, capitation, gatekeeper, utilization management, and health plan competition as cost containment strategies requires improvements in the tools used by quality review programs for detecting underprovision of appropriate health care services and poor outcomes of care. Otherwise, efforts to delegate responsibility, reduce micromanagement of practitioner and provider decisions, and encourage restraint in the use of resources may be accompanied by unwanted increases in immediate pain and suffering and long-term dysfunction. Oversight activities, however, tend to multiply rules, information requirements, and administrative costs.

The key criterion for judging the appropriateness of administrative tasks and costs is whether the costs they impose are justified by the degree to which they serve desired objectives related to access, quality, equity, efficiency, and information. The bases for evaluating claims in these areas are neither obvious nor settled among experts. Still, the committee believes that reform proposals ought to include clear and defensible statements about expectations concerning administrative costs and savings and the prospects for increased or decreased administrative burdens on patients and health care providers.

Tax Caps and Geographic Variations in Health Care Costs

A uniform national cap on the tax exclusion for employer-paid health benefits would likely be too generous for low-cost areas and a serious burden for many in high-cost areas. **The committee believes policymakers should provide for geographic indexing of any tax cap,** although it recognizes that this approach challenges the conventions of tax and benefit policy and could present significant technical and practical difficulties. If, however, the tax cap excluded some percentage of the cost of locally available health plans or if the tax cap were linked to the cost of the cheapest locally available health plan, then a form of geographic indexing would occur automatically.[2] Even if the details of

---

[2] The first option is analogous to the common employer practice of contributing 75 percent (or some other percentage) of the cost of the health plan chosen by the employee, with the employee paying the remainder.

an indexing strategy are left to administrative agencies, a reform proposal should provide basic guidance for their work. (In its discussion of access issues, the committee recommended that the supplemental coverage not be tax-favored unless the basic coverage is very narrowly defined.)

Patient Cost Sharing and Special Problems

As recommended earlier, requirements that individuals share in the cost of health coverage and health services should exempt some services (most notably, certain immunizations) and provide for some adjustment for low-income individuals within the bounds of administrative feasibility. Moreover, in addition to limits on annual out-of-pocket cost sharing, limits on multiyear out-of-pocket cost sharing should be defined to protect those with persistent health problems and high expenses year after year. Again, the details may be left to administrative agencies or perhaps a special commission, but a reform proposal should set forth basic criteria and procedures to be followed.

Core and Supplemental Benefits

In addition to provisions for patient cost-sharing, other decisions about the scope and depth of benefits will be strongly influenced by cost containment objectives. The committee has already recommended in its discussion of access that reform proposals should define a package of core benefits that health plans should cover and that proposals should allow consumers to purchase supplemental benefits under certain conditions. It has also noted the many technical and political questions and difficulties associated with turning such provisions into implementable policies and programs. To recapitulate, these questions and difficulties involve:

• the limits of available evidence about the health outcomes and costs of alternative forms of care for specific clinical problems and the consequent need for an incremental process of defining and updating coverage;

• the tensions between the desirability of a reasonably comprehensive benefit package and one that limits the cost of extending such coverage to those now uninsured;

• the problems of defining whether and what supplemental benefits should be permitted and the circumstances under which they might be, in part, tax-favored; and

• the multiple types of health plans (e.g., network and fee-for-service) that need to be considered in designing, implementing, and monitoring a benefits package and in establishing policies for supplemental coverage.

Risk Selection versus Cost Containment

As noted in the section on access, a health care reform proposal that relies on competition among health plans should discourage health plans from competing on the basis of risk selection rather than effective management of care and costs. **To promote the latter and limit the former, health care reform proposals should include provisions for standard benefit packages, risk-adjusted payments to health plans (but not risk-adjusted individual premiums), special provisions for very-high-risk individuals (e.g., reinsurance or separate risk pools), monitoring of marketing and other health plan practices, and similar measures (IOM, 1993b).**

CONTAINING HEALTH CARE COSTS

Key Statements

To serve health and access as well as cost containment objectives, policies to limit the rate of cost escalation need to be grounded in the concepts of:

• value—how health care spending relates to the achievement of desired outcomes;
• affordability—how health care spending relates to individual and societal resources; and
• equity—how the financing and distribution of health services affects different groups.

The committee did not formulate a comprehensive strategy to contain escalating health care costs in part, because evidence about the impact of such strategies is so limited.

The committee, however, agreed that several specific elements should have a role in a strategy for health care reform:

• Movement toward provider payment methods that encourage efficiency and economy in the provision of health services as well as quality of care and good outcomes
• Some cost-sharing by most patients
• Better information on the price, quality, and expected outcomes of medical services.

• Methods for quality and utilization review that help practitioners, patients, and others learn how actual care conforms to criteria for appropriate care and why care varies in effectiveness and efficiency

• A geographically indexed tax cap that limits the amount of employer-paid health benefits excluded from individual taxable income.

• Further movement to standardize many administrative practices and eliminate many costs associated with the immense diversity of current billing, payment, audit, reporting, and other practices.

The committee believes that reforms will require a pragmatic mix of regulatory and market strategies and that some degree of local flexibility and discretion is desirable.

Efforts to reduce administrative costs may, in some cases, conflict with efforts to collect more data for access and quality monitoring, educational, and other purposes. The key criterion for judging the appropriateness of administrative tasks and costs is whether the costs they impose are justified by the degree to which they serve desired objectives related to access, quality, equity, efficiency, and information.

To discourage health plans from competing on the basis of risk selection rather than effective management of care and costs, reform proposals should include provisions for standard benefit packages, risk-adjusted payments to health plans (but not risk-adjusted individual premiums), special provisions for very-high-risk individuals (e.g., reinsurance or separate risk pools), monitoring of marketing and other health plan practices, and similar measures.

Assuring the Quality of Care

To this point, the committee has had two key messages: (1) Health care reform proposals must aim to maintain and improve the health and well-being of the entire population, including groups with special health or access problems; and (2) reform planners must design and organize policies and programs to strengthen the value of health care expenditures—that is, what we can achieve, in terms of the health and well-being of individuals and populations, through health care spending. It has also stated that reform must be implemented so that expanding access and containing costs does not lead to unintended reductions in the quality of health care.

Reform plans can achieve these objectives only with explicit attention to quality, which includes defining, measuring, assuring, and improving the quality of care. Therefore, the committee proposes a set of quality-related principles and policies for health care reform proposals and advances an argument for greater attention to clinical practice guidelines.

By way of context, two major changes in medical care should be noted. First, care is being evaluated increasingly on the basis of its processes and outcomes, rather than on its structural aspects, such as the credentials of health care professionals. Second, with the advent of better research methods and computer technology, clinical medicine is becoming more science- and information-based. These two shifts should yield better and more cost-effective care in the future. In the committee's view, health policies and reform packages should not create incentives that retard these very positive and promising developments.

33

DEFINING QUALITY

Quality of health care has recently been defined by an IOM committee (1990h) as **the degree to which health services for individuals and populations increase the likelihood of desired health outcomes and are consistent with current professional knowledge.** The key concepts in this definition involve a broad view of health services; a focus on both individuals *and* populations; an expansive concept of health outcomes; a demonstrated link between processes of care (services) and outcomes; and an acknowledgment of the responsibilities of health professionals to stay abreast of their fields and to share with patients information about all reasonable alternative options in their care. This definition draws attention to a link between the processes of health care and the end results or outcomes of that care, in terms of both personal and social well-being and welfare. Additionally, it implies that individuals need to be well-informed about alternative health care interventions and their expected consequences (as well as about the expected damaging effects of decisions to pursue unhealthy lifestyles) and that, when making decisions about health care, clinicians need to take their patients' preferences and values into account.

Desired health outcomes are an especially important element for the quality-of-care dimensions of health reform proposals. **In considering such outcomes, reform proposals should provide for the use of a wide range of health-related quality of life measures; the array of tasks that might require such measures includes determining core benefits, assessing the effectiveness of health care technologies, and monitoring and improving the quality of care over time** (IOM, 1989c,f, 1990a,b,f,g,h; Lohr, 1989, 1992). The focus should not be on just the effect of health care on survival and life expectancy or various symptom, physiologic, and biologic states. Rather, quality assessment and assurance programs, and thus solid reform proposals, should also give attention to the impact on aspects of health that often matter most to patients, and about which they can give accurate reports; these include physical and cognitive functioning, role performance, emotional and mental well-being, and factors such as pain, energy, and vitality. Reform proposals should, finally, include measures of how people perceive their own health and of satisfaction with health care as important adjuncts to the outcomes related to health, functioning, and well-being. Proposals need not extend the scope of outcomes to the more expansive notions of quality of life. These involve the physical environment in which we live and work, the economic environment in which we labor, the skills we bring to coping with life's challenges, and the ethical, moral, and spiritual aspects of our lives. These factors, in many respects, are less appropriate as measures of health care outcomes than as indicators of circumstances that may limit or reinforce the impact of medical care.

QUALITY MEASUREMENT AND IMPROVEMENT

Simply asserting the benefits of quality assurance and improvement efforts will not suffice in an increasingly resource-constrained health care environment. To demonstrate the value of health spending, including spending for quality assurance and improvement activities to maintain high-quality health care services and good outcomes, reform proposals will need to proceed from several basic principles.

Major Targets

First, **reform plans should explicitly acknowledge three central issues that quality assurance and improvement efforts should address: (1) use of unnecessary or inappropriate care, as well as overprovision of otherwise appropriate services; (2) underuse of needed, effective, and appropriate care; and (3) lapses in technical and interpersonal aspects of care** (IOM, 1990h). These issues might be more simply characterized, respectively, as:

• "too much care"—the unnecessary or inappropriate care provided in this country costs money that could be put to more productive use and makes patients vulnerable to harmful side effects;
• "too little care"—necessary and appropriate services are often unused or unavailable, not only when people lacking health insurance delay seeking care or receive no care at all but also when even those

with insurance face geographic, cultural, attitudinal, or other barriers that limit their abilities to receive, for example, proper well-baby or well-child care, prenatal care, ongoing care for chronic illnesses, emergency care, rehabilitative services, or palliative care; and

• "inferior care"—health care professionals are expected to be able to diagnose and treat our ailments with competence and compassion, but not all clinicians have full mastery of their specialties, and not all can communicate with their patients with grace and empathy; these problems remain significant challenges to quality assurance and improvement efforts.

Criteria for a Strategy

Second, **proposals for reform should define an approach to quality assurance that will be meaningful, efficient, and acceptable to those with a stake in the process.** This includes patients and families, institutional providers and clinical practitioners, payers, and policymakers. For clinicians and patients, a participatory approach in which continuous improvement is the goal may be an important component of any quality assurance effort. One approach, for example, advances 15 criteria for judging the success of quality assurance or quality improvement programs (IOM, 1990h). It states that the program should:

• address poor technical or interpersonal quality, overuse of unnecessary or inappropriate services, and underuse of needed services;
• intrude only minimally into the patient–clinician relationship;
• be acceptable to health care professionals and provider organizations;
• foster improvement throughout the health care organization and system;
• identify and intervene to remedy demonstrably substandard performance (the so-called outlier or "bad apple" problem);
• invoke positive and negative incentives for change and improvement;

• provide well-motivated people with timely information to improve performance;

• possess face validity for the public and for professionals (i.e., be understandable and relevant to clinical decisionmaking);

• be scientifically rigorous (i.e., meet requirements for reliability, validity, and generalizability);

• improve patient well-being and outcomes in ways that can be measured and evaluated over time or that can be inferred from the process-of-care elements assessed;

• address both individual patient and population-based outcomes;

• document improvement in quality and progress toward excellence;

• be easily implemented and administered;

• be affordable and cost-effective; and

• include participation by patients and the public.

The committee recognizes, as did the original IOM committee for the Medicare study, that some of these attributes may be mutually exclusive and need to be traded off against each other. Furthermore, not all will be fully appropriate for different settings and types of practitioners or institutions, and in any case some cannot realistically be achieved in the short term. These are, nonetheless, the characteristics of a successful quality assurance and quality improvement effort toward which the system ought to move, even as reform plans are being put into effect.

Individual and System Perspectives

Third, the committee draws attention to the different perspectives that health care reform proposals need to reflect. On the one hand, **proposals will need to be concerned with the quality of care that individual plans and providers deliver**; this is a more traditional and familiar realm of assessing and improving the processes and outcomes of care given to individual patients and to persons enrolled in specific insurance programs. On the other, **proposals will need to attend to the quality of care across the entire system**, for instance, determining whether particular reforms do improve access to needed and appropriate services for all underserved populations.

Roles and Responsibilities

Fourth, **health care reform proposals must be clear about organizational structures, procedures, and divisions of responsibility and make explicit provisions for both internal and external monitoring of quality of care.** Specifically, they should set in place conditions that will help health organizations, provider groups, and practitioners act on their own to measure and improve quality. Two goals are sought. The first is to reinforce steps toward quality improvement at the local institution or plan level without introducing intrusive micromanagement programs from the outside; the second is to strengthen the performance of the system by rewarding exemplary performance and promoting continuous improvement of the average quality of care, not just by eliminating severely substandard practitioners or institutions. Reform plans will also need to involve existing or new regulatory programs to maintain outside surveillance on quality of care, and they may wish to provide for quality review activities by entities concerned with financing or consumer affairs. The committee wishes to emphasize, however, the importance of avoiding the external micromanagement of health care providers and of fostering self-evaluation, innovation, and internal quality improvement.

System Problems

Fifth, **the quality assurance and improvement program outlined in health reform proposals ought to include specific responsibilities for identifying and overcoming system and policy barriers to improved performance.** As suggested by the tenets of continuous quality improvement, wasteful and inefficient systems, as well as unduly complicated or contradictory policy environments, may contribute more to poor processes and outcomes of care than do the behaviors and practices of health professionals and institutions. The quality assurance efforts embodied in reform proposals should be designed to help surmount these problems, and they should do this in conjunction with the information-gathering efforts of stronger national surveys and the use of computer-based data files discussed in the section on infrastructure; progress will also depend somewhat on the generation of better evidence about the effects of practice guidelines on quality of care, as the evidence to date is preliminary and soft.

CLINICAL PRACTICE GUIDELINES

If advances in the nation's ability to measure and improve quality of care, as well as enhance value, are serious goals of reform, then proposals must explicitly endorse the development, dissemination, implementation, and evaluation of science-based guidelines for clinical practice. Clinical practice guidelines are "systematically developed statements to assist practitioner and patient decisions about appropriate health care for specific clinical circumstances" (IOM, 1990c; 1992b). The emphases in the IOM's view of guidelines are clear: assistance of clinician and patient decisionmaking, a focus on specific clinical circumstances, an insistence on systematic development, and an adherence to the best possible scientific base or, when data are not sufficient, the greatest possible consensus among health care professionals.

Practice guidelines are in a relatively embryonic state of development, especially insofar as cost containment, design of basic benefit packages, and other endeavors key to health care reform are concerned. Thus, as the committee has already suggested in its discussions of access and cost containment, health care reform proposals should not place more burdens on guidelines for solving problems of cost control, benefit package design, rationing, competition, administration, or quality than they, at their present stage of development, can sustain. Their emphasis should be on credible, accountable processes for developing and applying guidelines and, as noted in the Conclusion, on explicit support for the effectiveness and outcomes research needed to provide the scientific base for guidelines.

In the meantime, proposals can acknowledge that, with respect to quality assessment and assurance, thoughtfully designed and applied guidelines will help in four ways: (1) by improving patients' informed consent, their participation in decisionmaking, and their satisfaction with both the processes and outcomes of care; (2) by identifying important patient outcomes to incorporate in patient satisfaction surveys and other instruments designed to assess or improve performance; (3) by identifying possible quality problems arising from underuse, overuse, or incompetent provision of care; and (4) by determining priorities for improving or standardizing specific patterns of clinical care and sorting out competing claims for funding of biomedical and outcomes or effectiveness research. With respect to cost management, proposals can also recognize that those who pay for health care services and their agents can use guidelines in various ways, including (1) determining health insurance coverage and as screens to avoid paying for unnecessary or inappropriate care; (2) selecting or credentialing practitioners for participation in various health plans or institutions; and (3) tailoring other economic incentives to affect practitioner or patient behavior. The committee has, however, already cautioned against excessive expectations about the use of guidelines to control costs.

The IOM has proposed eight attributes by which the soundness of practice guidelines might be assessed and has developed a provisional assessment instrument based on those attributes (IOM, 1992b). Although judging the caliber of practice guidelines is not directly germane to health care reform, proposals ought to acknowledge that the quality of guidelines will be very relevant to quality measurement and improvement; consequently, the committee calls on reform advocates to provide for systematic evaluation of guidelines and similar tools, such as medical review criteria, that are produced in the coming years. Advances in this field will hinge, to some degree, on the headway made in related areas such as information systems and outcomes and effectiveness research, as discussed in the section on infrastructure.

SPECIFIC IMPLICATIONS

The committee's positions stated in the previous sections on access and cost containment have specific implications for the quality measurement and improvement program of any health care reform proposal. In particular, proposals should mandate that one responsibility of a quality assurance and improvement mechanism is to track health status and the use of services for identified, insured populations. Collectively, those populations will comprise all (or virtually all) people in this country.

Specific attention then needs to be given to services used (whether or not appropriate and necessary) and services *not* used that should have been (e.g., preventive care, prescription drugs). Note that the services not used that should have been cannot adequately be tracked by studying only those who use the health care system. Furthermore, special consideration must be directed at previously uninsured, vulnerable populations to see that appropriate outreach is mounted and that discrimination does not exist or persist.

Intersecting with these recommendations are those related to cost control. **The committee recommends that reform proposals mandate that a quality assurance and improvement program track the effects of certain cost containment processes.** This charge includes monitoring the impact of geographic global budgets and caps, if such are proposed. The aims are to ensure that necessary services are not curtailed excessively and that inappropriate queue-jumping does not occur. The charge also involves tracking the effects of increased use of health maintenance organizations, preferred provider organizations, and health insurance purchasing cooperatives that constrain the choice of physicians, other types of clinicians, hospitals, and the like. Such ongoing evaluation is necessary to be certain that continuity of care is not significantly eroded, that use of specialty care is not inappropriately restricted, and that outreach programs are maintained for special populations that face especially difficult barriers to access.

Finally, **a formal, nonjudicial mechanism by which individuals can voice grievances and obtain assistance should be available to all as the nation moves through the next few years of experimentation and change.** For example, even if certain reforms are enacted, such as amendments to the Employee Retirement Income Security Act (ERISA) and elimination of preexisting condition exclusions and waiting periods, situations may still arise in which certain kinds of plans may erect barriers to initial or continued health coverage or may link coverage in unacceptable ways to health status or social or demographic factors. These problems demand timely attention and resolution. Thus, **the committee recommends that health care reform proposals mandate an additional responsibility of a quality assurance and improvement program—namely, to serve as a focus for consumer complaints or as an ombudsman.** The committee does not envision the quality assurance mechanism suggested here as a substitute for reformed structures and processes to deal with patient allegations of malpractice.

Like access and cost containment, the commitment to quality of care—and the means by which it is assessed and improved—has implications for numerous other aspects of the health care system. For example, a common database (or common elements in multiple databases) able to track use and identify nonuse of services by enrolled populations will be needed; consequently, some provision needs to be made in reform proposals for defining and setting standards for databases that can be used in quality assessment and improvement programs.

ASSURING THE
QUALITY OF CARE

Key Statements

Reform plans should explicitly acknowledge three central issues that quality assurance and improvement efforts should address: (1) use of unnecessary or inappropriate care, as well as overprovision of otherwise appropriate services; (2) underuse of needed, effective, and (3) appropriate care; and lapses in technical and interpersonal aspects of care.

Proposals for reform should define an approach to quality assurance that will be meaningful, efficient, and acceptable to those with a stake in the process.

In considering outcomes, reform proposals should provide for the use of a wide range of health-related quality of life measures.

Reform proposals will need to reflect both concern with the quality of care provided by individual plans and practitioners and attention to the quality of care across the entire system.

Health care reform proposals should be clear about organizational structures, procedures, and divisions of responsibility and make explicit provisions for both internal and external monitoring of quality of care.

The quality assurance and improvement program outlined in health reform proposals ought to include specific responsibilities for identifying and overcoming system and policy barriers to improved performance.

Reform proposals should mandate that a quality assurance and improvement program track the effects of certain cost containment processes.

Practice guidelines are in a relatively embryonic state of development, especially insofar as cost containment, design of basic benefit packages, and other endeavors key to health care reform are concerned. Thus, as the committee as already suggested in its discussions of access and cost containment, health care reform proposals should not place more burdens on guidelines for solving problems of cost control, benefit package design, rationing, competition, administration, or quality than they, at their present stage of development, can sustain.

A formal, nonjudicial mechanism by which individuals can voice grievances and obtain assistance should be available to all as the nation moves through the next few years of experimentation and change. This committee recommends that health care reform proposals mandate an additional responsibility of a quality assurance and improvement program—namely, to serve as a focus for consumer complaints or as an ombudsman.

Financing Reform

Many steps proposed to improve access can be expected to add significant new financial burdens for employers, governments, and some individuals (e.g., those who moved from low-risk insurance pools to average-risk pools). Whether the nation will accept such burdens and how they will be distributed are clearly political decisions. As this report is being drafted, it is not clear that policymakers will feel they have sufficient popular support for the increased taxes that the committee expects will be necessary to protect more individuals against the financial consequences of ill health. Certainly, financing policies will be influenced by many considerations other than the equity, efficiency, and similar arguments identified in summary form by the committee. Again, this discussion does not constitute an IOM proposal for financing health care reform but rather is an attempt to identify issues and options.

Broad options for financing improved access for the uninsured and underinsured include:

- **reducing expenditures** on current health programs and services,
- **increasing the productivity** of the health care system,
- **shifting resources** from other areas of public spending, and
- **increasing revenues** from income, payroll, or other taxes or from individual insurance premium contributions.

These options are not necessarily mutually exclusive, and a combination of them is likely to be necessary. For instance, reductions in wasteful and excessive administrative spending could be expected to increase productivity as practitioners, managers, and others spend less time on paperwork and more time on patients. To cite another example, if some of the employer contribution to health insurance were treated as taxable individual income (as recommended earlier in this report), tax revenues would increase, although estimates of this increase vary depending on the assumptions about employer and employee responses. One desired effect of the change in tax policy is to reduce demand for generous health coverage, which would be expected, in turn, to reduce health services utilization and expenditures. The stronger this response, however, the less revenue might be expected from the tax cap, although that decrease would be offset to the extent that employers matched reduced health spending with higher wages as some economists would predict.[3]

In principle, the first step—cutting spending—may be achieved in many ways. The committee believes, however, that it is unrealistic to expect such good performance in reducing spending that all the costs of extending coverage could be offset, particularly in the short run. Given the great expansion in the share of national resources consumed by health care spending, it is also both unwise and unrealistic to argue that the nation can continue to draw resources away from other social objectives to the same degree it has in the past.

As a consequence, health care reform is likely to further burden financing arrangements that, in their current form, are often inequitable, inefficient, and poorly measured. For example, uncompensated care and underpayments by some public and private purchasers encourage crisis-oriented medical care, not prevention or timely therapeutic care, and they undermine the institutions that serve poor and vulnerable groups. Moreover, they increase costs for individuals and groups that lack the

---

[3]Tax caps are sometimes loosely grouped with several other kinds of financing strategies under the concept of means testing, whereby access to benefits is confined to certain categories of individuals (e.g., single mothers and their children) of limited means (i.e., income and assets). Medicaid is a classic example of a means-tested program. Although some have proposed that access to Medicare benefits should also be means-tested, more common—but still controversial—are proposals to link the beneficiary's share of the Part B premium (about 25 percent of the total) to income or to treat some of the government contribution to the Part B premium as taxable income.

political and economic leverage to protect themselves (IOM, 1993b). Many employers point out that their coverage of spouses subsidizes employers that do not offer coverage, and that cost-shifting associated with uncompensated care adds to this subsidy. To cite another example, the disparity in tax treatment of premiums for employed and self-employed individuals is inequitable and penalizes the self-employed. It may thereby promote overinsurance by the former and underinsurance by the latter.

Reform proposals should move the health care system toward more broad-based, efficient, equitable, and "observable" financing arrangements. They should be grounded in realistic estimates of expected expenditures and revenues and their distribution across population groups. Ad hoc efforts to compensate for overly optimistic forecasts tend to undermine program credibility and disrupt program stability. Likewise, inadequate recognition of how a proposal may affect different groups can create a "backlash," although the committee also recognizes that clarity about how burdens and benefits may be redistributed can compromise a proposal's chance of passage. The committee suggests that **the projections of revenues and expenditures be subjected to review and audit by independent, nongovernmental sources.**

To aid assessments of reform proposals, **the committee recommends that proposals for health care reform should explicitly:**

• **Describe anticipated sources of financing** (e.g., income taxes, payroll taxes, "sin" taxes, or a "tax cap" on employer-paid health benefits that can be excluded from personal income tax). The description should include estimates of revenues expected from each source (for multiple years) and the distribution of the financing burden across different income and other relevant groups.

• **Identify the expected level, distribution, and timing of savings expected from administrative reforms, cost containment strategies, infrastructure changes, and other provisions.**

• **Estimate the level and distribution of public and private expenditures (including tax expenditures) needed to implement the reform proposal over a period of several years.**

- State the assumptions, models, data, and similar elements used in developing the above estimates.
- Describe financing not only for health care services but also for basic elements of the health care infrastructure including public health, research, education, and capital investments.

Just as steps to increase access will add some costs so will certain steps to strengthen the infrastructure for the health care delivery system. Some of these steps, for example, improvements in our knowledge about the impact of medical services and our spending for these services, may increase short-term costs but provide the basis for longer term savings. Others may only improve the quality of care, thereby providing better value without actually reducing costs. In the next section we discuss infrastructure issues that should be covered by proposals for health care reform.

FINANCING REFORM

Key Statements

Reform proposals should move the health care system toward more broad-based, efficient, equitable, and "observable" financing arrangements. They should be grounded in realistic estimates of expected expenditures and revenues and their distribution across population groups.

Proposals for health care reform should explicitly:

• describe anticipated sources of financing.

• identify the expected level, distribution, and timing of savings expected from administrative reforms, cost containment strategies, infrastructure changes, and other provisions.

• estimate the level and distribution of public and private expenditures (including tax expenditures) needed to implement the reform proposal over a period of several years.

• state the assumptions, models, data, and similar elements used in developing the above estimates.

• describe financing not only for health care services but also for basic elements of the health care infrastructure including public health, research, education, and capital investments.

Projections of revenues and expenditures should be subjected to review and audit by independent, nongovernment sources.

Improving the Infrastructure for
Effective Change

Making policy is not the same as implementing it. The necessary conditions for effective short- and long-term implementation of a proposal for health care reform should be considered in the design of the proposal. Some of the conditions for successful change involve matters beyond the scope of a reform proposal per se, for example, political leadership and the general condition of the economy. Reform proposals should, however, discuss how certain broad features of the governmental and health care delivery infrastructure will be designed or shaped to support the objectives of reform. Four important elements of this infrastructure are:

• **governance and administration,** which involve the transformation of statutes into regulations, enforcement and oversight mechanisms, and other public and private actions needed to implement reforms;
• **human and physical capital,** which includes the appropriate level, mix, and distribution of health care professionals, facilities, and equipment;
• **knowledge development,** that is, the biomedical, clinical, and health services research and the health data systems that create, aggregate, analyze, and disseminate information that practitioners, administrators, consumers, and others need to continuously improve health and meet other objectives of reform; and

• **public health policies and programs** that focus on the community rather than on the personal health services that are the central concern of health care reform.

In addition, other elements may be considered part of the administrative apparatus necessary to promote the goals of health care reform in the longer run or to advance other important social goals. Among these are, for example, the definition of clinical malpractice, the creation of better legal responses to clinical errors, and the protection of the privacy and confidentiality of sensitive patient data that reside in computer-based records and databases.

GOVERNANCE AND ADMINISTRATION

Different reform proposals involve vastly different and difficult-to-catalog levels and distributions of governance and administrative responsibilities. The committee does not take a position on the "ideal" administrative structure for health care reform; that structure must be fitted to the specifics of a particular proposal. **Whatever the specifics, however, reform proposals should be clear about the roles, responsibilities, accountabilities, and interrelationships of the public and private sectors in implementing the proposal and achieving its objectives.** Proposals should define explicitly:

• the program management responsibilities that will reside in the public sector and the level of government—federal, state, local, or some combination—that should discharge them;
• the administrative tasks to be undertaken by private sector entities such as employers, fiscal intermediaries, or health care providers; and
• the role, if any, of quasi-public organizations such as a commission or board that might define covered services or certify health plans for which public enrollment subsidies would be available.

Most reform proposals will probably require some reorganization of the Department of Health and Human Services to accommodate new responsibilities and realign existing activities. The nature of this reorganization will necessarily differ for different plans, and many details may properly be worked out subsequent to the adoption of reform legislation. Nonetheless, the basic assignment of planning, operational, oversight, and evaluative tasks needs some preliminary definition. As one example, a federal role in quality monitoring and improvement may call for the creation of a new entity or agency that can address quality-of-care problems and promote quality improvement activities for the entire age range covered by the health plans (i.e., not just the elderly covered by the Medicare program's Peer Review Organization effort).

All reform proposals should provide for greater standardization and efficiency in some administrative tasks. This should be simpler for some proposals, for example, those that call for automatic enrollment (e.g., at birth) in a single national health plan. Proposals that incorporate competitive health plans will have to identify how much uniformity and simplicity is desirable and feasible with respect to such matters as criteria or rules for monitoring the quality and appropriateness of services, tracking eligibility for coverage under different health plans, filing claims for payment, reporting information on outcomes, and using electronic data interchange technologies. The Workgroup for Electronic Data Interchange (1992) has recommended that such computerized capabilities be adopted by all insurers, employers, and providers. The IOM has urged reductions in the intrusive and disruptive micromanagement of clinical practice that now prevails through many utilization management programs (IOM, 1989b). The committee endorses the principles and aims of these earlier groups.

Although some short-term costs will likely be incurred in achieving greater uniformity, simplicity, and efficiency in program administration, costs should be reduced over time. Frustration with the system should also decrease among most affected parties—patients, clinicians, and administrators. The criterion for judging the appropriateness of whatever administrative tasks—and thus costs—remain is the degree to which they serve desired objectives related to access, quality, equity, efficiency, and information. The bases for evaluating claims in these areas are not obvious or agreed upon by experts, but the committee believes that reform proposals ought to have some clear and defensible statements about expectations concerning administrative costs and savings.

Beyond these statements, the administrative implications of different reform proposals and the need for program specifications vary so much that only examples will be given of the kinds of administrative issues that should be covered in reform proposals. For instance, reform proposals that envision negotiations between physicians and payers over payment for medical services probably will require adjustments in antitrust policies, as well as guidelines and rules for the negotiation process and its outcomes, and should specify who would make decisions if negotiations fail.

To cite another example, some reform proposals may call for certain services to be provided through regional institutions such as designated transplantation centers, shock-trauma units, and neonatal and pediatric intensive care units. Proposals for such regionalization should be as specific as possible about what services might be regionalized (if that is known) or what criteria and processes would be used to identify such services, as well as about how such institutions will be identified, certified or designated, and recertified. Some delegation of decisionmaking to the states might, for example, be explicitly anticipated.

Virtually no observers of the health care scene believe that reform can be or will be instantaneous. Rather, many elements of reform will have to be phased in, and some steps may have to be contingent on the outcomes of earlier changes. **The committee recommends that reform proposals be clear and realistic about the timetable expected for full implementation. Moreover, monitoring mechanisms will be needed to detect inadequate implementation, unanticipated negative effects, and positive results that should be built upon.** The full details of the timetable for implementation may emerge as the initial stages of the implementation move forward, but the reform plan should reflect careful consideration of the phasing of implementation—those aspects that are essential first steps and those that will require the development of new tools and programs. The monitoring and evaluation efforts will be essential elements of the phasing, and clear responsibilities for such long-term monitoring and research should be described. Ongoing program evaluation, although expensive and time consuming, provides the knowledge to determine whether we are moving in the directions sought through health care reform and to make appropriate mid-course corrections in policies or their implementation.

HUMAN AND PHYSICAL CAPITAL

In extending health insurance coverage and pursuing serious cost containment, health care reform, regardless of its form, will shape the demand for and distribution of human and physical capital. This shaping may be unintended (as, for example, was the impact of initial Medicare reimbursement policies on hospital capital financing and on the relative incomes of physicians by specialty). Alternatively, the reform plan can include deliberate steps to ensure that human and physical capital support reform goals. A variety of mechanisms currently direct the flow of capital resources: market forces heavily influenced by reimbursement policies of payers in the public and private sectors, public and private regulations, and specific investment policies. Many actors—public and private—have determined these policies.

Another characteristic of decisions about capital is their long-term impact. The training of a physician takes many years; a hospital facility will last decades. Thus, steps taken today can be expected to have effects a quarter-century from now.

Because a health care reform plan is unlikely to replace totally this configuration of factors affecting capital, the committee believes that it is critical for the reform plan to give explicit attention to both health personnel and physical capital policies that connect these important long-term inputs to the desired objectives of the reform plan. This attention should deal with at least the following:

- reimbursement policies that shape the market forces driving many human resource and physical capital decisions made by individuals and institutions;
- policies that provide direct investment in capital, such as support of health professions education and public sector support for capital plants and equipment;
- policies for the distribution of highly specialized, capital-intensive services for which distribution by market forces alone may not be desirable;
- regulatory policies that affect the supply, distribution, and roles of health personnel; and

• policies that affect the development and introduction into practice of new technologies and procedures that will help form the human and physical capital requirements of the future.

Without taking a stand on the nature of the policies, **the committee recommends that any plan should make clear how it will deal with issues of human and physical capital supply and distribution.** The plan need not specify detailed approaches to all of these issues. It should indicate, at least, a process by which policies will be established and effects of the reform plan on capital will be monitored so that policies can evolve in support of the plan's goals. The reform plan's objectives must be congruent with the long-term development of health personnel and physical capital. The plan should consider the establishment of an ongoing commission, or other equivalent mechanisms, that can ensure this congruence of policies as the plan evolves, monitor results, and make the necessary mid-course corrections.

The committee also notes that health care reform plans calling for major reconfigurations of arrangements for services, such as the creation of new health care plans providing comprehensive services, will generate up-front capital requirements to pay for the costs of the necessary consolidations and reorganizations of providers. These initial investments in organizational capital will need to be financed out of the future stream of revenue.

Human Capital

Several prominent proposals for health care reform emphasize primary care providers and their role as the managers, coordinators, or gatekeepers of health care services for patients. This stance presupposes an adequate supply of primary care physicians and other practitioners, such as nurse practitioners and physician assistants. This assumed supply does not match either today's mix of specialists and generalists or the mix projected to emerge in the next several years from today's professional training programs. In the short run, therefore, such reform proposals must be clear as to how the proposed system will actually function, given the current supply of primary care physicians.

("Current" in this context implies through roughly the year 2010.) In the longer run, attention will need to be directed at determining "what the right numbers are" for generalists and specialists and how the relevant education and training programs will be supported.

The committee recommends that health care reform proposals describe policies and priorities that determine the role of various providers, including nurses and physicians, and the settings from which they should deliver care. Particular emphasis must be given **to primary care providers and how the shortfall in such clinical disciplines can be overcome both in the near term and over the longer run through changes in practitioner payment methods, educational programs, and improvements in the attractiveness of the primary care function.**

Significant changes in the pattern of financing may leave certain types of health professions education and training vulnerable to underfunding, possibly graduate medical and nursing education in particular. Conversely, reform also creates opportunities for effecting desired changes in health professions education (as implied above concerning primary care), and these opportunities should be identified and seized even in the early years of reform.

A number of IOM reports have dealt with the need to strengthen primary care (1978, 1984a,b), nursing and nursing education (1983), future directions for the allied health professions (1989a), and support of graduate medical education in ambulatory settings (1989d). Most of these reports discuss the important correlation between the methods and patterns of health care financing and the training and deployment of health personnel. Those designing health reform packages should take account of these well-known relationships in contemplating how the reimbursement of plans, networks, purchasing cooperatives, facilities, and free-standing practitioners (e.g., physicians or nurse practitioners) might be managed to achieve more appropriate incentives for the cost-effective deployment of human resources and supportive educational and retraining strategies. Since much of the support for the education and training of health personnel is derived from the financing of patient care, changes in the patterns of that financing will need to give specific attention to adequate financing of educational programs appropriate for the reform strategy. The financing can be included in or separated from

the financing of patient care.   Since much of the support for the
education and training of health personnel is derived from the financing
of patient care, changes in the patterns of that financing will need to give
specific attention to adequate financing of educational programs
appropriate for the reform strategy. The financing can be included in or
separated from the financing of patient care.

Physical Capital

Through the years, the United States has wavered between varied,
and sometimes conflicting, policies concerning the supply and
distribution of physical capital. Direct public investment (e.g., the Hill-
Burton program), state and regional planning (voluntary or enforced
through certificate of need), and market forces responding to
reimbursement policies have all been used. A health care reform plan
should be explicit about how it will influence investment in physical
plants and equipment to be consistent with the fundamental goals of
access, efficiency, and quality. The plan will need to be concerned, at
the least, with the geographic distribution of services (including
regionalization of highly specialized services), reduction of unneeded
capacity or redistribution of existing capacity, response to new
technologies, the needs of particular populations such as the elderly and
the urban poor, replacement of aging physical plants, and the capital
requirements for teaching and research. The plan will need to deal with
the locus of decisionmaking for these varied needs and with the mix of
policies that balance long-term needs with shorter term responses to
changing requirements.

KNOWLEDGE DEVELOPMENT

Databases, Surveys, and Information Technologies

Successful implementation of health care reform will require more
and better data and information about health care, especially in the face
of the pressures that can be expected as a new system tries to hold down

expenditures while expanding access and maintaining high-quality care. Health care providers, patients, the public, and policymakers all will be asked to make harder and more complex choices and trade-offs than in the past. Informed choices dictate a vastly increased need for improved data and information for operations, evaluation, and research.

As a case in point, defining and refining an appropriate package of basic benefits would present a stiff challenge even with far more information than we have today about the efficacy and effectiveness of health care services.[4] Similarly, a comprehensive quality assurance system will require a greatly enhanced database on the use of services, patient outcomes, and the processes of care. The creation of these kinds of databases, only the foundations of which currently exist, will be a major undertaking. **The committee recommends, therefore, that reform proposals include a specific mandate for the development and continued support of comprehensive health databases.** These should contain material on access to and availability of care, use of health services and technologies, outcomes of care, demographic information, and information on health plans. These data can be used in health services, effectiveness, and outcomes research, technology assessments, and the evaluation of national and state health care reform efforts.

From the time of the first national census in 1790, an important role of the federal government has been to provide objective statistical data to inform and guide decisions and social policies in a free society. In light of the rapid changes in health care now occurring and the prospect of further dramatic change, this federal responsibility becomes even more acute, and it intersects significantly with the previous recommendations concerning research, data, and databases. **The committee recommends taking steps to improve the nation's survey and statistics capabilities, particularly by instituting a national health care survey that can**

---

[4]The distinction between efficacy and effectiveness is important. Efficacy is typically defined as the outcome of an intervention when it is applied in "ideal" circumstances, such as those in prospective randomized clinical trials; this is the purview, for instance, of much of the research agenda of the National Institutes of Health. In contrast, effectiveness refers to the outcome of an intervention when applied in the daily practice of medicine to the medical problems of typical patients; research in this area is supported chiefly by the Agency for Health Care Policy and Research.

track progress and identify problems in the implementation of reform efforts.

The National Center for Health Statistics has proposed an innovative national survey intended to greatly improve our knowledge about the functioning of the health care system. In *Toward a National Health Care Survey: A Data System for the 21st Century* (NRC/IOM, 1992b), a joint IOM/NRC committee suggested ways to make this survey an even better source of data about the use and effects of health services—for example, patterns of care, the cost of care, health status and other characteristics of individuals receiving care, and the demand for and use of services over time and across a broad range of providers and service settings.

National survey data would complement information derived from health care operations, such as insurance claim forms and hospital discharge abstracts; these sources typically are the core of the kinds of health databases discussed above. National survey data would also supplement information that, in the future, may be derived from computer-based patient records (CPRs) and CPR systems.

In a recent report, *The Computer-based Patient Record: An Essential Technology for Health Care*, an IOM panel explored the problems of today's patient records, which are still predominantly paper based, and the opportunities afforded by a shift to computer-based systems (IOM, 1991b). Universal adoption of CPRs promises all the following: better patient information to support clinical decisions; improved management of care by making quality assurance procedures and clinical practice guidelines more accessible to health care professionals at the time and site of patient care; reduced administrative costs; and more relevant, accurate data necessary for provider and consumer education, technology assessment, health services research, and related work concerning the appropriateness, effectiveness, and outcome of care. **The committee recommends that reform proposals promote universal implementation of CPRs and CPR systems among providers.** Complete development and adoption of CPRs will be a lengthy and challenging task. Although progress is being made, explicit commitment in health care reform proposals in this area will provide a further impetus to complete this technological and behavioral revolution and to use information and electronic technologies as a lever for progress in controlling costs, expanding access, and improving quality.

To promote related advances in information services and technologies, **the committee also recommends adoption of an expanded program in information services for health services research and technology assessment at the National Library of Medicine (NLM)**. Recent legislation requires the NLM to improve its array of services; to do this, the library has undertaken various developmental efforts in the areas of vocabulary, indexing, and management of databases and other information resources.

An IOM committee asked to review NLM activities and plans made several recommendations related to the library's long-term goals (IOM, 1991e). The recommendations involve improving access (including automated access) to a wide range of published and other information important to those who deliver health care and to those who produce and use health services research; promoting use of the NLM's information services by a wider range of audiences and interest groups than has heretofore been the case; and expanding and enhancing the traditional reference, research assistance, coding, and retrieval activities of the library and its national network of libraries. Although the committee does not expect reform proposals to deal with these information technology and services issues in detail, it does express its hope that the need for and utility of the NLM's broad scope of activities will be recognized and supported at least in general terms.

Privacy and Confidentiality of Sensitive Personal Health Data

Increasingly, concerns about the privacy and confidentiality of sensitive health data are drawing the attention of providers, patient and consumer groups, legal experts, ethicists, and computer specialists (IOM, 1991b, 1993b; Workgroup for Electronic Data Interchange, 1992). Reform plans that rely heavily on health-related, patient-identified information in large databases must acknowledge the social, legal, and ethical problems inherent in these issues and, ideally, propose some steps to protect patients' privacy rights. These safeguards must be strong (and must be perceived to be strong), but they should not interfere with appropriately approved research and system evaluations of the types discussed above.

Health Services, Outcomes, and Effectiveness Research

In the health sector, many different types of basic and applied research are needed, and sophisticated biomedical and clinical investigations have long been a hallmark of the research enterprise in this nation. To assure the continued flow of new knowledge about health and disease that will be the basis for more definitive preventive and curative strategies, the remarkable record of biomedical research productivity needs to be sustained. With respect to the looming changes in health care delivery that reform promises, however, greater attention will have to be given to the clinical evaluation sciences, including outcome and effectiveness research, and to health services research. To provide this knowledge and analytic base, **the committee recommends an absolute increase in the support for a range of research and information activities that should be carried out if reform is to be implemented and evaluated satisfactorily, particularly in the areas of clinical evaluation sciences and health services research.**

Several IOM committees have addressed the promises and limitations of research on effectiveness and outcomes in health care (1989c, 1990a,b,e,f). Among the key aspects of effectiveness research are generating accurate, valid, and reliable data; following patients over time and across settings of care; comparing alternative approaches to care; and tracking a broad range of patient-relevant outcomes including self-reported quality of life and health status (Lohr, 1989, 1992). The expansion of the medical effectiveness program of the Agency for Health Care Policy and Research (created in late 1989) was an important step in expanding research on effectiveness and outcomes.

Effectiveness research complements the biomedical research that is the scientific substrate of both clinical medicine and clinical epidemiology, which emphasizes the incidence and prevalence of disease. It adds an important dimension to these efforts by helping physicians and other health professionals, patients, the public, and policymakers better understand what can be expected from alternative courses of care, a key requirement for making determinations about value. Therefore, adequate support of effectiveness research, as well as biomedical research, is a necessary and integral part of any health care reform plan that hopes to improve the value received for our investments in health care.

Health services research might be said to comprise a focus on the health status of individuals, populations, or both; review or analysis of health systems, health interventions, and the factors that influence health status; a comprehensive set of variables involving health care techniques, practices, programs, and policies; and the combination and integration of these variables in many ways, frequently emphasizing the nonbiological aspects of health and medical care (IOM, 1991e; see also IOM, 1979). From this listing, the relevance, if not the absolute necessity, of health services research should be clear.

The committee believes that reform proposals serious about self-evaluation will make support for such a research agenda a high priority.[5] Some proposals, but by no means all, explicitly address issues of quality of care, for instance by suggesting the creation of a national program of quality assurance. Others may directly or indirectly call for efforts at technology assessment, development and application of clinical practice guidelines, and various consumer education and outreach activities. Still others advocate various changes in the nation's approach to malpractice liability (e.g., tort reform as a piece of the larger reform picture). All these matters are within the health services research purview. The committee believes that among the specific areas deserving attention are quality measurement, assurance, and improvement (IOM, 1990h; 1991f) and clinical practice guidelines issues, particularly with respect to techniques of development, methods of dissemination and application, and evaluation (IOM, 1990d, 1992b). Research in selected topics such as aging (IOM, 1991d) and disability prevention (IOM, 1991c) will also be important. Therefore, for purposes of informing the full range of

---

[5]Examples of the questions that reform proposals generate in the area of *health services research* include: How will reforms affect access to care by different subgroups of those currently insured and uninsured? How will reforms affect total spending on health care, the rate of increase in expenditures, and specific factors that influence spending (e.g., new technology, and the purchase of less generous health coverage)? If a spending cap is adopted, will it work as expected? Will financing mechanisms work as anticipated with respect to their adequacy and as to their effect on the distribution of the financing burden? What unanticipated consequences may also emerge? What major problems with health care will the public and policymakers identify?

health care reform efforts over the ensuing decade, a sustained investment in general health services research equivalent to that for effectiveness research, if not for biomedical research, will be needed.

Technology Assessment

Hand in hand with clinical evaluation and health services research, as well as biomedical research, go health technology innovation and assessment. Changes secondary to health care reform are expected to affect the use of existing technologies (e.g., through the development of basic benefit packages) as well as to influence the extent and direction of technological innovation. For these reasons, **the committee recommends that steps be taken to improve the nation's capacity to execute effective technology assessments and that reform proposals be explicit about how they will deal with the innovation and diffusion of health technologies**. Questions about the impact of cost containment on the innovation, development, and diffusion of medical technologies can be expected to arise, so ideally reform packages ought to anticipate these issues even if they cannot at this early stage propose definitive plans for managing technological innovation and change (IOM, 1991g, 1992c). Given the scarce resources available in the public sector for technology assessment, mechanisms for setting priorities for technology assessment deserve attention (IOM, 1992f). Finally, as is true for the development of practice guidelines, quality criteria, and similar informational, educational, administrative, or evaluative tools, some efforts will need to be directed at developing better methods to establish a consensus about good (or poor) health care practices and to carry out appropriate studies of the costs and benefits (i.e., the value) of health care services (IOM, 1990d,g; 1991a).

PUBLIC HEALTH POLICIES
AND PROGRAMS

Health care reform is understandably focused on issues relating to personal health care services. The committee recognizes that many factors that affect the health of the population (e.g., air and water pollution, personal behaviors affecting health, and protection against personal injury) have a primary locus external to the direct delivery of personal health services. The committee strongly urges that reform proposals explicitly recognize the need for support of the public health sector. In *The Future of Public Health*, an IOM committee advanced numerous recommendations for strengthening the mission of public health—namely, "fulfilling society's interest in assuring conditions in which people can be healthy" (IOM, 1988, p. 7)—and overcoming the disarray of public health. These recommendations dealt both with structural aspects of public health, including the governmental role in public health and types of responsibility at the federal, state, and local government levels, and with organizational focal points for public health, special linkages (to, for instance, environmental health, mental health, and care for the indigent), strategies for capacity building, and education for public health.

A partnership between the personal health services system and the population-based activities of the public health system, as well as occupational health activities, should be encouraged in the reform proposal. This partnership is essential for dealing with many significant health issues, such as AIDS, resistant strains of tuberculosis, unhealthy dietary practices, substance abuse, case-finding and outreach, and emergency services. By explicitly recognizing these important links, the reform proposal can avoid the unintended starvation of public health programs in the competition with health care reform for scarce public funds.

OTHER INFRASTRUCTURE ISSUES

Programs for Special Populations

The earlier discussion of access noted that the needs of special populations may require targeted public programs. It also emphasized that the role of existing public programs, in particular, Medicare for the elderly and disabled and Medicaid for some of the poor, will have to be defined. These are infrastructure as well as access issues.

Tort Reform

It is hard for the committee to conceive of successful health care reform over the long run that does not address the real and perceived problems related to our current system for dealing with medical liability for bad clinical outcomes.

Reform proposals should, at a minimum, acknowledge these problems and either define general directions for tort reform or specify a process and timetable for defining such directions and translating them into specific policy proposals. This committee, however, lacked the resources to define those directions as they relate to changes in tort law, adoption of alternative structures for dispute resolution, and similar options. The discussion below highlights points raised in IOM reports on quality of care and clinical practice guidelines.

A major criticism of the current system for determining medical liability is that it is not a reliable vehicle for screening out or rejecting unwarranted claims of malpractice. The consequences of this unreliability include high malpractice insurance costs, psychological burdens on practitioners, higher health care costs stemming from "defensive medicine" (i.e., care that would not be provided but for the fear of litigation), and even incentives for practitioners to abandon certain kinds of medical practice (e.g., obstetrics). Less prominent in much of the discussion of tort reform is the criticism that the current system leaves much malpractice unidentified and unremedied (IOM, 1991g). Tort reform efforts should acknowledge both criticisms of the current system and should recognize the role of quality assurance programs and other vehicles for responding to elements of these criticisms.

First, improved programs of quality assurance and continuous improvement can do much to detect performance problems, identify their causes, and develop administrative and clinical strategies for improving performance and avoiding future problems (IOM, 1990h, 1991g). A preventive approach clearly has advantages over after-the-fact compensation of victims, although the latter is also appropriate.

Second, the grievance process recommended in the preceding section of this report may deflect some unwarranted claims of malpractice. It may also lead to acceptable resolution of some real cases of malpractice without the expense and trauma of a trial.

Third, clinical practice guidelines have a role to play in efforts to reduce the incidence of malpractice and to resolve specific claims of medical liability (IOM, 1991g). Some guidelines may target specific sources of malpractice suits (e.g., anesthesia-related injuries). In the context of changing judicial views of the appropriate standard of care, guidelines may help judges and juries better identify bad outcomes due to substandard care. Further, guidelines formulated to help patients better understand the likely benefits and risks associated with treatment alternatives may reduce litigation inspired by poor communication and disappointment resulting from unrealistic hopes. However, another IOM study committee has concluded that it was premature to endorse state legislation granting practitioners immunity from liability if they have practiced in accord with guidelines developed at legislative behest (IOM, 1991g). The committee was concerned about weaknesses in the processes for developing such guidelines and assessing their soundness. It also believed that plaintiffs as well as defendants should be able to cite robust guidelines in their arguments.

Malpractice and tort reform are complex issues that perhaps need not be woven directly into health care reform from the outset, although some committee members thought otherwise. The options for malpractice and tort reform go far beyond the points we have discussed above. These options include statutory reforms (such as barriers to suits or reductions in damage awards), arbitration and mediation as alternatives to litigation, no-fault approaches, various kinds of administrative programs that may involve disciplinary (fault-based) actions (like those now in theory done through licensure boards), so-called early offers of settlement (done on a voluntary basis by offending providers and practitioners), mechanisms based on private contracts between providers and patients, and enterprise liability (in which institutions such as hospitals, health plans, or others undertake to cover individual practitioners in malpractice situations). Little or no empirical evidence suggests which of these strategies might be effective in which situations, and hybrid arrangements might also be possible. The committee believes that reform proposals should, at a minimum, acknowledge the need for change and perhaps indicate what strategies would appear to mesh best with the type of reforms envisioned.

Public/Consumer Education

Although reform proposals vary in their emphasis on the consumer as an informed purchaser of care or the patient as an informed decisionmaker about courses of treatment, the proposals share a common infrastructure requirement: more extensive and effective public and patient education programs and tools. Market-oriented reforms require explicit attention to the kinds of comparative information provided to individual purchasers of health plans, the source and accuracy of that information, and its real utility. The conditions for effective consumer decisionmaking may also include other changes discussed in this and other IOM reports, for example, some standardization of benefit design and regulation of health plan marketing practices.

To educate individuals faced with making decisions about possible courses of care for specific medical problems, clinical practice guidelines that consider outcomes relevant to patients and variations in patient preferences for different types of care and outcomes can—in the form of practitioner guidelines—help physicians and other health care practitioners better educate patients and—in the form of patient guidelines—help directly build patient understanding. New educational media such as the interactive video disc technology may at the same time standardize the information provided to patients and increase its relevance.

IMPROVING THE INFRASTRUCTURE FOR EFFECTIVE CHANGE

Key Statements

Reform proposals should be clear about the roles, responsibilities, accountabilities, and interrelationships of the public and private sectors in implementing the proposal and achieving its objectives. All reform proposals should provide for greater standardization and efficiency in some administrative tasks.

Reform packages should be clear and realistic about the time-table expected for full implementation. Monitoring mechanisms will be needed to detect inadequate implementa-tion, unanticipated negative effects, and positive results that should be built upon.

Any plan should make clear how it will deal with issues of human and physical capital supply and distribution.

Health care reform proposals should describe policies and priorities that determine the role of various providers, including nurses and physicians, and the settings from which they should deliver care. Particular emphasis must be given to primary care providers and how the shortfall in such clinical disciplines can be overcome both in the near term and over the longer run through changes in practitioner payment methods, educational programs, and improvements in the attractiveness of the primary care function.

Reform proposals should include a specific mandate for the development and continued support of comprehensive data-bases in the health field.

The committee recommends taking steps to improve the nation's survey and statistics capabilities, particularly by instituting a national health care survey that can track progress and identify problems in the implementation of reform efforts.

Reform proposals should promote universal implementation of computer-based patient records (CPRs) and CPR systems among providers. The committee also recommends adoption of an expanded program in information services for health services research and technology assessment at the National Library of Medicine.

The committee recommends an absolute increase in the support for a range of research and information activities that must be carried forth if reform activities are to be implemented and evaluated satisfactorily, particularly in the area of clinical evaluation sciences and health services research.

The committee recommends that certain steps be taken to improve the nation's capacity to carry out effective technology assessment efforts and that reform proposals be explicit about how they will deal with the innovation and diffusion of health technologies over time.

A partnership between the personal health services system and the population-based activities of the public health system, as well as occupational health activities, should be encouraged in the reform proposal.

Conclusion

Constraining the rapid escalation of health care costs while extending health insurance coverage to all—the primary objectives of health care reform—will require significant improvements in the performance of our system for health care. This performance imperative is especially important because some of the factors behind rising health care expenditures, such as the aging of the population, are external to the health care system.

In the Preamble to this report, we set forth the committee's view that the fundamental goals of reform are to maintain and improve health and well-being, to make basic health coverage universal, and to encourage the efficient use of limited resources. The preceding sections of this document have provided a broad framework for assessing whether and how different reform proposals would pursue these goals. The elements of that framework—extending access to health care, containing health care costs, assuring quality of care, financing reform, and improving the infrastructure for effective change—all need to be addressed if system performance is truly to be improved. In some areas, we have made specific substantive recommendations based on the work of other IOM committees or the clear consensus of this committee; in other areas, we have laid out questions that proposals should answer.

A long-term perspective is essential. A framework for assessing reform, such as that we have suggested, will be useful both for the initial evaluation of proposals and for the assessment of progress over time. Indeed, to be most useful, as the results of reform efforts unfold the

71

committee's recommendations should be subject to the same type of ongoing evaluation as the reforms themselves.

The complexity of the health care system—and of health itself—presents major challenges to reform, and these challenges are intensified by the many important and often contending interests that have a stake in both the broad directions and intricate details of policy change. Reform proposals that focus primarily on financial issues and goals without recognizing that improved performance requires significant changes in how health care is organized and provided are unlikely to achieve the goals outlined here. Reform proposals must indicate their general approach to questions such as how health care professionals are to be appropriately trained and deployed (including expected responses to market signals from revised incentives), how better information is to be marshalled to improve performance, and how quality of care can be maintained and improved within resource constraints.

Finally, the reform of our health care system should be undertaken in the same spirit of continuous improvement and renewal that has so often been the keystone of success in America. The profound changes required for effective reform, even when the nation builds on the existing strengths of its health care system, demand that we learn from experience. To do that we need good information and sound analyses of results, flexibility and creativity in responding to that information, and an abiding focus on the concerns of the people whose health and well-being we seek to improve.

References

CBO (Congressional Budget Office). *The Effects of Managed Care on Use and Costs of Health Services.* Washington, D.C.: U.S. Government Printing Office, 1992a.

CBO. *The Potential of Direct Expenditure Limits to Control Health Care Spending.* Washington, D.C.: U.S. Government Printing Office, 1992b.

EBRI (Employee Benefit Research Institute). *Issues in Health Care Cost Management.* Washington, D.C. Issue Brief Number 118, 1991.

IOM (Institute of Medicine). *A Manpower Policy for Primary Health Care.* Washington, D.C.: National Academy of Sciences, 1978.

IOM. *Health Services Research.* Washington, D.C.: National Academy of Sciences, 1979.

IOM. *Nursing and Nursing Education: Public Policies and Private Actions.* Washington, D.C.: National Academy Press, 1983.

IOM. *Community Oriented Primary Care: A Practical Assessment. Volume One: Report of A Study.* Washington, D.C.: National Academy of Sciences, 1984a.

IOM. *Community Oriented Primary Care: A Practical Assessment. Volume Two: Case Studies.* Washington, D.C.: National Academy of Sciences, 1984b.

IOM. *Preventing Low Birthweight.* Washington, D.C.: National Academy Press, 1985.

IOM. *The Future of Public Health.* Washington, D.C.: National Academy Press, 1988.

73

IOM. *Allied Health Services: Avoiding Crises.* Washington, D.C.: National Academy Press, 1989a.

IOM. *Controlling Costs and Changing Patient Care? The Role of Utilization Management.* B.F. Gray and M.J. Field, eds. Washington, D.C.: National Academy Press, 1989b.

IOM. *Effectiveness Initiative: Setting Priorities for Clinical Conditions.* Washington, D.C.: National Academy Press, 1989c.

IOM. *Primary Care Physicians: Financing Their GME in Ambulatory Settings.* Washington, D.C.: National Academy Press, 1989d.

IOM. *Quality of Life and Technology Assessment.* F. Mosteller and J. Falotico-Taylor, eds. Washington, D.C.: National Academy Press, 1989f.

IOM. *Acute Myocardial Infarction: Setting Priorities for Effectiveness Research.* P. Mattingly and K.N. Lohr, eds. Washington, D.C.: National Academy Press, 1990a.

IOM. *Breast Cancer: Setting Priorities for Effectiveness Research.* K.N. Lohr, ed. Washington, D.C.: National Academy Press, 1990b.

IOM. *Clinical Practice Guidelines: Directions for a New Program.* M.J. Field and K.N. Lohr, eds. Washington, D.C.: National Academy Press, 1990c.

IOM. *Consensus Development at the NIH: Improving the Program.* Washington, D.C.: National Academy Press, 1990d.

IOM. *Effectiveness and Outcomes in Health Care. Proceedings of a Conference.* K.A. Heithoff and K.N. Lohr, eds. Washington, D.C.: National Academy Press, 1990e.

IOM. *Hip Fracture: Setting Priorities for Effectiveness Research.* K.A. Heithoff and K.N. Lohr, eds. Washington, D.C.: National Academy Press, 1990f.

IOM. *Improving Consensus Development for Health Technology Assessment: An International Perspective.* Washington, D.C.: National Academy Press, 1990g.

IOM. *Medicare: A Strategy for Quality Assurance* (2 Vols.). K.N. Lohr, ed. Washington, D.C.: National Academy Press, 1990h.

IOM. *The Artificial Heart: Prototypes, Policies, and Patients.* J. R. Hogness and M. VanAntwerp, eds. Washington, D.C.: National Academy Press, 1991a.

IOM. *The Computer-based Patient Record: An Essential Technology for Health Care*. R. Dick and E.B. Steen, eds. Washington, D.C.: National Academy Press, 1991b.

IOM. *Disability in America: Toward a National Agenda for Prevention*. A.M. Pope and A.R. Tarlov, eds. Washington, D.C.: National Academy Press, 1991c.

IOM. *Extending Life, Enhancing Life. A National Research Agenda on Aging*. E.T. Lonergan, ed. Washington, D.C.: National Academy Press, 1991d.

IOM. *Improving Information Services for Health Services Researchers. A Report to the National Library of Medicine*. J. Harris-Wehling and L.C. Morris, eds. Washington, D.C.: National Academy Press, 1991e.

IOM. *Kidney Failure and the Federal Government*. R.A. Rettig and N.G. Levinsky, eds. Washington, D.C.: National Academy Press, 1991f.

IOM. *Medical Innovation at the Crossroads. Vol. II. The Changing Economics of Medical Technology*. A.C. Gelijns and E.A. Halm, eds. Washington, D.C.: National Academy Press, 1991g.

IOM. *Guidelines for Clinical Practice: From Development to Use*. M.J. Field and K.N. Lohr, eds. Washington, D.C.: National Academy Press, 1992b.

IOM. *Medical Innovation at the Crossroads. Vol. III. Technology and Health Care in an Era of Limits*. A.C. Gelijns, ed. Washington, D.C.: National Academy Press, 1992c.

IOM. *Nutrition During Pregnancy and Lactation. An Implementation Guide*. Washington, D.C.: National Academy Press, 1992d.

IOM. *Nutrition Services in Perinatal Care* (2nd ed.). Washington, D.C.: National Academy Press, 1992e.

IOM. *Setting Priorities for Health Technology Assessment. A Model Process*. M.S. Donaldson and H.C. Sox, Jr., eds. Washington, D.C.: National Academy Press, 1992f.

IOM. *Access to Health Care in America*. M. Millman, ed. Washington, D.C.: National Academy Press, 1993a.

IOM. *Employment and Health Benefits: A Connection at Risk.* M.J. Field and H.T. Shapiro, eds. Washington, D.C.: National Academy Press, 1993b.

Jencks, S., and Scheiber, G. Containing U.S. Health Care Costs: What Bullet to Bite? *Health Care Financing Review* 1991 Annual Suppl.:1–12, 1991.

Lohr, K.N., guest ed. Advances in Health Status Assessment: Conference Proceedings. *Medical Care* 27(March Suppl.):S1–S294, 1989.

Lohr, K.N., guest ed. Advances in Health Status Assessment: Fostering the Application of Health Status Measures in Clinical Settings. *Medical Care* 30(May Suppl.):MS1–MS294, 1992.

Newhouse, J.P., Manning, W.G., et al. Adjusting Capitation Rates Using Objective Health Measures and Prior Utilization. *Health Care Financing Review* 10(3):41–54, 1989.

Newhouse, J.P. Medical Care Costs: How Much Welfare Loss? *Journal of Economic Perspectives* 6(3):2–21, 1992.

NRC/IOM. *Including Children and Pregnant Women in Health Care Reform: Summary of Two Workshops.* S. Brown, ed. Washington, D.C.: National Academy Press, 1992.

NRC/IOM (National Research Council). *Toward a National Health Care Survey: A Data System for the 21st Century.* Washington, D.C.: National Academy Press, 1992.

Thorpe, K. Health Care Cost Containment: Results and Lessons from the Past 20 Years. In: *Improving Health Policy Management: Nine Critical Research Issues for the 1990s.* S.M. Shortell and U.E. Reinhardt, eds. Ann Arbor, Mich.: Health Administration Press, 1992, pp. 227–274.

Workgroup for Electronic Data Interchange. *Report to Secretary of U.S. Department of Health and Human Services.* Washington, D.C.: U.S. Department of Health and Human Services, 1992.